The Art of American Health Care

Peter Q Warinner, M.D.

For my fellow medical doctors and our patients

Contents

Preface

I consider this book my testimony regarding the state of health care in America today. It presents my opinions based on real-world hands-on professional experience. It does not reflect the positions of any academic institution, any business entity or any professional organization that I am currently or formerly affiliated with. I know there are many doctors and patients that share these opinions but their voices remain unheard or suppressed. I estimate it is the overwhelming majority of doctors and patients that share most of these opinions.

I do not present myself as THE expert on the subject matter, but I consider myself AN expert on the subject matter from the perspective of a clinical allopathic medical doctor and surgeon on the front lines of patient care.

The essence of my testimony is that the implementation of health care in America today has abandoned its historic focus on the protection of the doctor-patient relationship and replaced it with a focus on centralized control over health care money and medical decision making – now with the doctor and the patient being the last or least considered in every aspect of health care.

In spite of this dire situation, there is still a chance to save the American health care system. As I dissect through and expose many of the serious flaws, I also propose innovative solutions to heal the damage.

Doctors and patients, armed with the following information, stand up and demand change. Act now to preserve, protect and prioritize the doctor-patient relationship with a focus on what is best for the doctor and what is best for the patient in the American health care system of the future. Help make the American health care system great again. Act now because very soon it will be too late.

Peter Q Warinner, M.D.

Chapter One:

What Do Patients Want?

1. In a fantasy world, patients want medical doctors and technology to be able to perform miracles. If a medical issue arises, a patient wants to see a medical doctor immediately. He wants that doctor to be fully competent, kind, attentive and respectful. He wants that doctor to spend as much time as necessary to solve that problem then and there. He wants that doctor to have devices, right there in the office, that can make the correct diagnosis, treat the medical issue and put everything back to normal by the end of the day.

2. Patients want to be seen in a timely fashion commensurate with the urgency and severity of their problem. Patients want doctors to be on time and spend a reasonable amount of time with them during the encounter. Patients understand that doctors have other patients and other time commitments, but their time is valuable too and their medical problem must be reasonably addressed.

3. Patients want their medical doctors to look at them, listen to them, believe them, respect them, honor their privacy, guard their vulnerabilities and focus on them during the encounter without being distracted. Patients want their doctors to be mature, wise, compassionate, honest, professional and personable but not too personal. Patients want to feel safe from harm, safe from abuse and safe from being taken advantage of in any way.

4. Patients want their medical doctors to be competent and reasonably comprehensive. Patients want their medical doctors to be minimally intrusive and minimally invasive. Patients do not want specialists and subspecialists and sub-subspecialists; they want a doctor that can see the big picture and take care of them rather than referring them to many other doctors each of whom will assess only one tiny aspect of the big picture and otherwise be useless. Patients may not be able to avoid specialists, but the trend toward ever increasing sub-sub specialization must be reversed because it lowers quality of patient care, even though it might be intellectually stimulating to a doctor.

5. Patients want their medical doctors to engage with them directly. It would constitute a superior patient experience to have students and trainees as apprentices and assistants serving with the doctor at his side, instead of as substitutes attempting to serve in place of the doctor. Patients want their medical doctors to communicate with them using language they can understand, to provide education and to be reasonably accessible after the encounter.

6. Hospital and emergency room patients want to tell their story only once or twice – not seven or ten or however many more times. The current practice of having the patient tell the story first to the triage nurse, then to the treating nurse, then to the medical student, then to the intern, then to the resident, then to the chief resident, then to the fellow, then to the attending doctor, then to the specialist and other consultants is maddening and leads to mistakes and poor quality care and loss of confidence in care, yet this is the current standard of care.

7. Patients want health care costs to be reasonable and not wasteful. Patients want to be able to afford health care or at least

2

have an effective insurance plan to cover the costs. Patients want their medical doctors and medical facilities to be paid appropriately and in a timely fashion.

8. Some patients don't want to take personal responsibility. Imagine the common scenario whereby a patient has recovered from a heart attack. This patient suffers from morbid obesity, muscle weakness due to sedentary deconditioning (sits all day), consumes alcohol daily, consumes caffeine daily, smokes multiple cigarettes daily, smokes marijuana, has type two diabetes and has been instructed by his doctor numerous times to quit smoking, quit substance abuse, lose weight, modify diet, exercise and take medications as prescribed. The patient is continuously non-compliant and so has another heart attack. The doctor would not have had to treat the first or second heart attack if the patient would have taken responsibility for his own actions, for his own lifestyle and for his own health. This is a form of self-destructive behavior, suicidality. From a certain perspective, this patient's doctor may be considered a failure since he was unsuccessful in helping the patient to make the necessary changes.

9. Sometimes what patients want from medical doctors is unreasonable or even unlawful. It is common for patients to request that doctors fraudulently fill out documents so that the patient can receive disability benefits or workers compensation benefits or a handicap placard for their car or prescriptions for controlled substances for black market resale, etc. If the doctor refuses to comply, such patients usually go "doctor-shopping," meaning that they will go from doctor to doctor until they find one that will fulfill their request. However, sometimes such patients will threaten the doctor to coerce his cooperation. The threats can be of physical violence or of filing a "complaint" with

the board of medicine in the state (fabricating a lie about the doctor's inappropriate behavior). More commonly, threats can be of going to a physician-rating website to write a scathing review. Clearly, no doctor should give in to such bullying or unlawful behavior; however, most doctors remain entirely unsupported in defense of such actions. There is no state board of patients to report to, there are no patient rating websites, and to call police or to file a lawsuit every time this occurs is unsustainable.

10. I propose a patient's oath:

I hereby vow to treat my doctor with respect and authority commensurate with the doctor's level of training and licensing. I vow to comply with all instructions and prescriptions provided to me by my doctor. I vow to alert my doctor to any problems with my ability to comply. I vow that if, for whatever reason, I cannot comply with my doctor's instructions and prescriptions, after sincere effort, and after the doctor's attempts at modifications, then I will seek care from a different doctor. I vow not to threaten or manipulate my doctor to perform some action against my doctor's free will. I vow not to deceive my doctor. I vow not to attack my doctor either verbally or physically or otherwise harm my doctor openly or secretly. I vow to compensate my doctor according to our pre-agreed payment plan. I understand that my doctor is a fellow human being who has normal human flaws and did not give me my illness or injury. I understand that my doctor is limited by the current flaws of medical knowledge and the current flaws of medical technology. I understand that my doctor is bound by local, state and federal laws and regulations.

Chapter Two:

A Medical Doctor's Oath

I propose a new, more comprehensive, contemporary Medical Doctor's Oath. This can be broadened as a Clinician's Oath and it can be customized to other specific health care clinicians. I instruct all medical doctors to print this out, sign it, display it, and live by it.

A Medical Doctor's Oath

I vow to treat each patient as an individual human being; I will not define any patient as a disease or an injury or a diagnosis. I vow to practice the arts of medicine and surgery limited by my knowledge, training, experience, laws and authority. I vow to be honest about my own limitations and defer to a more experienced medical doctor when necessary and if possible.

I vow to maintain a holistic approach to understand each patient within the context of family, local culture, regional environment, religion, academic achievement, athletic involvement, vocational influences and social structure.

I vow to spend sufficient time with my patients, to look at them, to listen to them, to effectively communicate with them, to honor their privacy, to guard their vulnerabilities, to be sincere in my pursuit of their best interests, and to do no harm.

The Art of American Health Care

I vow to care for each patient free from the influence of any political, religious, academic, commercial or financial bias or conflict of interest. I vow to prioritize my efforts for the benefit of my patients above the benefit of my career, my academic affiliation, my research project, my business entity, my employer or my government.

I vow to care for each patient free from prejudice against any aspect of gender, race, ethnicity, religion, intellectual ability, age, income level, criminal status, political affiliation, substance addiction, medical diagnosis or lifestyle choices. I vow to keep all aspects of my patient's health care information private and share only what is required by law or what the patient instructs me to share.

I vow to conduct myself in a professional manner at all times with every patient, never taking advantage of any patient in any way, especially considering ways of a financial or carnal nature. I vow to maintain a clean and healthy lifestyle.

I vow to continually seek further education in the arts and sciences of medicine and surgery while ever improving my understanding of human nature. I vow that as I gain knowledge and experience, to the best of my ability, I will add to the repertoire of services I provide to my patients rather than limit the services due to personal interest. I vow to learn practical business skills so I will be able to serve my patients free from outside influences.

I vow to remain committed to my patients, my community and my society to preserve the health of the health care system. I vow to be active on local, regional, state, national and international levels, to the best of my ability, to prevent third parties from taking over control of, or interfering with, the doctor-patient relationship.

I vow that on the day I become physically or mentally unfit to perform my duties as a medical doctor, or on the day I cease to agree with any one of these vows, that will be the day I conclude my career as a medical doctor.

Chapter Three:

The State of the Art of Medicine

1. The practice of "western medicine" or "traditional medicine" or "conventional medicine," better categorized as allopathic medicine, contrary to popular belief, is not an exact science. It must incorporate science plus the intangible skill of healing through human interaction. The skill of a medical-doctor-healer may be based on scientific knowledge regarding human anatomy and physiology and pharmacology, but that merely sets the stage on which healing can take place. The human body itself is capable of self-repair and self-healing under the right circumstances. The art of medicine requires the medical doctor to have the appropriate scientific knowledge and technological skill. It requires the medical doctor to have a mature and wise understanding of human nature. It requires the medical doctor to combine these attributes during meaningful encounters customized to each unique patient.

An honest assessment of the state of the art of clinical medical care in America today (or on Earth today) is that we are still in the dark ages. Teams of academics, entrepreneurs and politicians, who poorly understand human sickness and wellness, compete amongst themselves to control the health care system. Relatively primitive processes and methods are kept in place. They oppressively inhibit innovation in order to preserve third-party profits and preserve a feudalistic system. Individual human lives might be prolonged, but quality of life and efficacy of care are of little concern. One hundred years into our future, people will look back at this time and remark how medieval our health care system was.

Patients must understand that most medical knowledge today is opinion, based on interpretation of scientific data, combined with empirical experience, and is not fact. It is a misconception that medical knowledge is fact and that doctors are interchangeable because they are just implementing textbook facts. Given one patient and a list of seven symptoms, ten doctors may suspect five different diagnoses. Given the same diagnosis, ten doctors may propose twelve different treatment plans.

In spite of these flaws, most patients ultimately do well because of the tremendous power of the human body to heal itself, most often regardless of what the doctor does or doesn't do. Hence, the greatest principle that guides doctors' actions is to do no harm. If the doctor does something for the patient, it might help. If the doctor does nothing for the patient, it still might help. If the doctor harms the patient, it is usually due to the perilousness of the patient's condition in spite of the doctor's efforts to help, combined with the limitations of current medical knowledge and technology. On some occasions the harm is due to human error which is an unavoidable aspect of life. On rare occasions the harm is due to malicious intent which may be considered criminal.

2. A medical doctor exclusively adopting a scientific approach may have some success following one-size-fits-all algorithmic recipes for diagnosis and treatment of disease states and injuries; however, the success may be partial or short-lived. If the issue is a simple one, such as a simple bacterial infection requiring a specific antibiotic prescription, then the scientist may be able to handle it entirely with scientific methods.

3. A non-medical-doctor "alternative" practitioner might have the skill to gain the patient's confidence and may help the patient to feel better, but will ultimately fail, in cases of true medical illness or injury, because the practitioner's "knowledge" may be faulty or even dangerous. If the issue is a simple one, such as a simple stomachache from fear of public speaking, then the "alternative" practitioner may be able to handle it entirely.

4. Human patients are often considered all the same on the inside: tubes, muscles, blood, bones, nerves and fluids – comparable structures and mechanisms from patient to patient with minor differences. So the prevailing theory in the medical community is that if we can compile the right algorithms, then we wouldn't need medical doctors anymore. The theorists envision that someday a patient will be able to itemize his symptoms into a computer program, then the program will figure out the diagnosis and treatment plan. If surgery is necessary, then a robot will be programed to do the surgery. Proponents of this vision are the dominant thought shapers in the medical world today. However, their thought processes are faulty because humans are not all the same. Currently, many people are turning to the internet, trying to use it like this envisioned program. The internet doesn't work that way: it cannot diagnose you and it might interfere with your treatment because your search results will bring you fear, confusion and anxiety instead of appropriate knowledge.

5. When medical doctor scientists do clinical research and publish articles regarding patient care, and their colleagues cite such articles as recipes to diagnose and treat their patients, this behavior is absurd and potentially harmful. Every clinical research study has inclusion criteria, exclusion criteria and

multifactorial issues that make the results applicable only to a certain percentage of those in the study. The resulting information and conclusions can NOT be applied to any one individual patient, especially one that does not meet all the inclusion and exclusion criteria, or one that is unique in any way compared to those in the study (and that's just about everybody). Additionally, no study ever shows conclusion 100 % unanimous in favor of one course of action. However, tragically, such research has been used as the foundation of what is known as "evidence-based medicine." It is comparable to religious dogma. Medical doctor scientists use this "evidence" to develop algorithms and guidelines and protocols to diagnose and treat individual patients. Whereas it was once left to the judgment of the individual clinical medical doctor, considering his individual patient, to decide what is best.

It is now forced on doctors to obey such algorithms and guidelines and protocols – regardless of patient outcomes. Medical doctors are even being told that if they follow the guidelines, and the outcome is poor, then it is not their fault. Conversely, they are being told that if they do not follow the guidelines, even though the outcome is good, then they will be reprimanded and punished. Medical doctors are being brainwashed into institutional obedience rather than fighting to maintain the capacity for independent thought.

What is worse is that said algorithms and guidelines and protocols are being developed by health care organizations, insurance companies and governmental bodies often with clinical medical doctors playing little or no role.

The statistical analysis that is done related to the raw data in many medical research studies may be manipulated. Take into consideration that medical research studies are promoted (published) or suppressed (not published) based on subjective issues, such as who has influence and control over that academic facility or over that professional journal – not necessarily based on the merits of the study. Considering all of this, then the concept of "evidence-based-medicine," as it is practiced today, is a farce. Additionally, the concept of using algorithms or guidelines or protocols, as it is practiced today, is a farce.

6. Medical doctors of today are often more focused on distractions than on becoming healers. During their training many choose the easiest options at every stage so that they can appear more impressive – rather than choosing the most difficult pathways to test their resolve and develop clinical strength. They focus on passing multiple choice tests – rather than on expanding their knowledge or clinical experience. They focus on social media and social life – rather than on selflessly and anonymously immersing their existence into the depths of the human condition. They focus on convenience – rather than on service. They focus on appearances – rather than on substance. They focus on research – rather than on patient care. They focus on themselves and their career self-promotion – rather than on their patients and their community. I'm not describing all medical doctors, but I am describing an disturbing trend compared to the past. The art of medicine is a dying art.

7. Medical doctor healers additionally must understand that a patient does not become ill or injured in a vacuum – it usually occurs within the complex social context of family and peers. A full understanding of the diagnosis and optimal efficacy of the treatment plan cannot be accomplished unless the social

dynamics are tactfully elicited, confidentially understood and creatively incorporated into the plan.

8. During my training I was once told by a mentor that patients are not to be treated as friends in any way. It was an announcement he made to all trainees in the group, and I suspect he announced this to group after group for many years. I disagreed with that statement then, and I still disagree with it. It is important for the medical doctor to perceive the patient as a friend, a neighbor, a family member. Granted, in order to be most effective, a successful medical doctor must be able to detach himself from the patient and suppress emotions which could interfere with performance and cloud judgment. No patient will do well if the medical doctor treats him as if he is an object on an assembly line. At the same time, a medical doctor who becomes too "friendly" with a patient crosses the line of professionalism. A successful medical doctor healer must master this social balance.

9. All health care is local. To think that some bureaucrats in Washington D.C. should be entitled to decide what is best for all medical doctors and for all patients across the country – micromanaging from the greatest distance imaginable, with the greatest conflict of interest and the greatest invasion of privacy – is a nightmare scenario that has been brought into reality. This cancerous process invading the American health care system must be halted and expunged.

The medical doctor healer needs to fully understand the state or region or community in which he practices. He needs to know the history and the people. He needs to know the local culture, folklore, customs, unique beliefs and mindsets. He needs to know the local infections, toxins, hazards, climate and geography. He needs to know the local laws and policies. He needs to understand the individual patient within this context.

10. Medical doctor healers must serve their communities as well as their patients. A community maintains a sense of confidence when it can recruit and maintain quality medical doctor healers who provide consistent, trustworthy, reliable, quality health care services to the patients of that community for years and decades – often across generations of families. A community that experiences a high turnover of medical doctors is an unstable and unhealthy community. Medical doctor healers must keep this in mind and make a commitment to a community for the long run and forego moving from place to place even if they believe it will somehow elevate their careers.

Chapter Four:

Obstacles to Patients Receiving Quality Care

1. Ever increasing cost of health care. Health care costs are increasing due to unbridled profits authorized to pharmaceutical companies and biomedical technology companies and hospital entities by governmental agencies and insurance companies based on lobbying and negotiating success. It is a myth that medical doctors make obscene profits and are to blame for the rising costs. The truth is that the sum of all medical doctors' net personal income represents a relatively tiny percentage of the total costs in the American health care system (some estimates calculate it at less than 0.5%). Doctors' real income, adjusting for inflation and expenses, has been diminishing every year for decades.   However, governmental agencies and insurance companies focus each year on further reducing doctors' real income knowing that doctors have little to no power to stop them.

Patients must understand that the money spent to pay for their health care insurance does not go to the doctor. Patients must understand that the payment their insurance company makes to the doctor after a doctor's visit is not the doctor's personal income – it is a payment to cover all of the expenses in the doctor's office. A small percentage is actually left over for the doctor's personal income. If the payment is made within the context of a hospital visit, almost none of that payment will be for doctor's income. Doctor's incomes in the 1970s and 1980s might have been lucrative, but far from it anymore. At this time, doctor's personal income is severely limited and tightly regulated, but salaries and profits for hospital administrators, pharmaceutical company employees and biomedical technology company employees are obscene and unchecked. I know of pharmaceutical sales representatives (some with no more than a high school degree) who make much higher personal income than medical doctors. Many hospital administrators (who are non M.D.s) can make income five or ten fold what a doctor in their hospital makes – even at "non-profit" hospitals.

Pharmaceutical companies, biomedical technology companies, major hospital organizations and the like may have tremendous cash hoards and employ armies of attorneys and lobbyists to get what they want out of favorable governmental and commercial policies and payment schemes. The doctors and the patients don't stand a chance against this kind of financial and litigative and legislative muscle.

With the recent radical changes in health care laws, with the random annual unreasonable changes in the Medicare system and with commercial health care insurance companies apparently exempt from anti-collusion regulations, costs to the patients have been rapidly rising year after year. There is the increased cost for the health care insurance policy. There is the increased deductible. There is the increased copay. There is the increased cost of medications that the insurance policies refuse to cover. The overall trend is to pay the doctors less, force the patient to pay more, increase the profits for the health care insurance companies, increase the profits for the pharmaceutical companies, increase the profits for the biomedical technology companies, and increase the pay for the hospital administrators.

2. Patients being treated by physician extenders. This phrase has come to refer to clinical health care providers that are not medical doctors, but supposedly work under the direction and supervision of medical doctors. This refers to Nurse Practitioners [N.P.s] and Physician Assistants [P.A.s].

When N.P.s and P.A.s work closely with medical doctors and are well trained and experienced in that doctor's practice (far beyond their initial training for their degree), then the quality may be quite good. However, due to faulty ideas and ignorant legislation, in some states and regions, N.P.s and P.A.s are inadequately trained and inappropriately allowed to practice allopathic medicine independently from medical doctors.

The faulty ideas include the theory that N.P.s and P.A.s can handle most common and simple things and so the medical doctor can be spared for the more difficult and complicated things. This is faulty because if the common and simple things are not handled with wisdom and appropriate expertise, then they quickly become more difficult and complicated, alternatively, sometimes things that appear common and simple to the untrained eye are actually more difficult and complicated.

3. Incompetent or underutilized doctors. Medical doctors are less competent today than in recent past decades. Doctors are rewarded far less these days for their efforts, and so fewer intelligent successful people are attracted to the field. These days, at each stage of filtering, doctors are less likely to be chosen for their chances of success or for their clinical skill, but chosen for their likelihood to comply with undue outside influence. In

the past, doctors were chosen for their potential for excellence regardless of gender or skin color or other discriminatory factors. However, today, at each stage of filtering, doctors are chosen to fill contrived quotas of gender, skin color, ethnicity, etc. Leadership roles within the medical hierarchy are filled not by competence, but based on docility or friendship connections or religion. The most skillful doctors are usually not chosen for leadership roles because those in command do not want people who are smarter or more talented to threaten their authority or supremacy. In the health care hierarchy today, it is considered preferable to have influence and control over information and people rather than to empower quality and excellence.

Needlessly handicapped by the current misguided health care system, primary care doctors and emergency room doctors – arguably the most important doctors in the health care system – are sometimes relegated to the role of triage nurse. Triage is the concept whereby patients are separated by the level of seriousness and urgency. Traditionally this has been decided by a so skilled nurse, and the nurse would then refer the patient to this doctor or that and decide who needs to go immediately and who can wait. Today when a patient goes to a primary care physician, rather than diagnose and treat the patient, that physician often will send the patient to a specialist – this underutilizes the primary care doctor. Likewise, in many emergency rooms today, a patient will be seen by the emergency room physician only to be told that a specialist consultant is needed to diagnose and treat the patient – this underutilizes the emergency room doctor. Patients would be better served if primary care doctors and emergency room doctors could structure their practices to provide services at greater depth and breadth.

4. Specialists, subspecialist and sub-subspecialists. Imagine a medical doctor that has such a narrow focus that he will only see patients that have an injury involving one nerve in the left pinky finger – and he will see no other patients. Furthermore, if the patient he is seeing with that circumscribed problem has other health issues, he will not address them. This may seem like nonsense, but it actually occurs, especially at the academic medical centers. What a waste of human resources, what a waste of a medical degree and what a waste of a medical license. Patients would be better served if specialists would not forsake their roles as general medical doctors for the sake of personal trivial pursuits. Their pursuits of knowing more and more about less and less must be in addition to, not instead of, their practice of general medicine.

5. Academic facilities. Academic facilities are best known as the famous medical centers that are affiliated with medical schools and residency training programs and also known as teaching hospitals. These facilities usually spend exorbitant amounts of money on propaganda public relations efforts to convince the local and regional communities that they provide state of the art cutting edge medicine and surgery and that their doctors are the thought leaders of medical science, etc., blah, blah, blah. These facilities concentrate similar efforts brainwashing their employees and students and trainees that the facility is the greatest place in the known universe for anyone and everyone to get their health care, and if anyone is getting their health care anywhere else, their life might be in danger. In many cases, with few exceptions, the inside secret is that the famous academic

teaching hospital environment is one of the worst places to get health care. It is best to avoid academic teaching hospitals, if possible, and instead go to local private practice medical doctor offices and smaller community hospitals. That is where you are more likely to get the best expertise and quality of care. This is why I have moved my practice away from the large academic hospital setting, away from any hospital setting, into the community setting – for the benefit of my patients.

At the famous academic teaching hospital, whether as an outpatient or as an inpatient, your care will be provided by, and led by, students and trainees and academic/scientist/researcher-type doctors that typically have poor clinical ability. So much time may be wasted. So many unnecessary tests may be ordered (often not even the correct tests). Care may be so much more expensive. Care may be of much lower quality. The chance for misdiagnosis may be high. The chance for inappropriate or even harmful treatments or procedures may be high. You may have to wait many months for follow up care and you may wind up seeing a different doctor and trainee every time.

It is almost comical, if it weren't so serious, when I see the scenario of the person who demands to be seen only at the most famous academic teaching hospital by only the most famous researcher chairman full professor doctor. Sometimes there is the lack of understanding that the famous researcher academic doctor does not spend the bulk of his time actually taking care of patients, and so he will be rusty in the art of clinical care (with outdated knowledge because he has not been keeping up with anything other than his miniscule area of lab rat research). Sometimes, there is also the lack of understanding that the doctor who is designated as chief of service or chairman of the department is often chosen due to his political maneuvering and administrative collaboration with hospital administrators, not because of his clinical skill.

Patients need to choose a doctor, not a hospital or a medical center or health care organization. I know the patient may be bound for a poor outcome when I hear them say something to the following effect: "I need to go to The Greatstone General Hospital at Best School Medical University so I can get the best care possible." Conveyed in this statement is the common misconception that the famous place will cure the person by virtue of its fame, when, ironically, the opposite is more likely.

One solution for the waste and low quality care and high costs within the context of the academic medical center teaching hospitals is that Medicare and all commercial insurers must be entitled to a cost differential lower reimbursement to the facility and doctors when care is provided within that environment. Today the opposite is true.

I will go further to state that doctors should only be paid or reimbursed for patients that they see or treat directly, without the proxy of medical students or residents or fellows. If there is an academic encounter whereby a medical student or resident or fellow is involved, then the reimbursement should be to that student, resident or fellow and the payment should go toward the cost of his education and training. Furthermore, contrary to how it is now, the federal and state government should not be paying for the training of residents. The way it works now is that the government pays the academic medical center a large sum of money annually for each trainee (intern and resident), and the trainee receives a fraction of that as their salary (for the substantial work they do), and the academic medical center keeps the remainder, less expenses, as profit.

6. Hospital-based imaging. As a medical doctor, when I order an MRI test for a patient, I try to avoid hospital-based imaging centers. As an example, when I order a brain MRI at a private stand-alone MRI center outside of a hospital facility, the cost might be in the range of $1,000 – $1,500. When I order the same image at a community hospital, the cost might be in the range of $2,500 - $3,500. When I order the same image at an academic medical center, the cost might be in the range of $4,500 - $6,500. Ironically, when doctors, who are employed by, or affiliated with, said community hospitals or academic medical centers, try to send their patients "outside" to the lower cost facility, they will be reprimanded and even financially penalized in some cases. This is a maneuver such facilities employ to discourage "leakage." Leakage is loosely defined as health care dollars being spent outside of the financial benefit of a particular organization, even if it is for the sake of higher quality patient care and lower overall health care costs. This concept can be expanded to include any hospital-based procedure that could otherwise be completed more cost effectively outside the hospital.

7. Being trapped in a health care organization. With each passing year, increasing numbers of medical doctors are being forced out of private practice settings into hospital employed settings. This represents an influential and dangerous but hidden and secret conflict of interest. These doctors are no longer serving the patients. They are serving the hospital corporation, the academic institute, the government – essentially they serve some health care organization and not the patient. These doctors are rewarded when they engage in behavior that benefits the

supremacy and control and financial well-being of the health care organization. Likewise, they are punished if they do anything to the contrary – regardless of the impact on the patient. Rather than use independent judgment about diagnostic or treatment decisions (based on their education, training, skill and care for the patient) they will follow diagnostic and treatment algorithms, guidelines and protocols developed by administrators and lawyers and financial consultants at the health care organization or by government.

In cases where a patient might benefit from the expertise of a specialist who works outside of a particular health care organization, the referring physician who works inside that health care organization is prohibited from sending the patient to that specialist and must send the patient to a specialist "within the organization" even if it is the wrong match. The same goes for any test or procedure. If the patient or the doctor do not cooperate, then each of them will be threatened with various penalties, including financial. This new culture causes doctors to view other doctors, who work "outside" their particular health care system, as enemies.

Many states have what is known as certificate of need [CON] regulations which protect established hospitals and prevent potential competitors from building new facilities (such as new hospitals, surgical centers and imaging centers). This government-sanctioned restriction of trade further empowers establishment hospitals to impose their will on any given community.

Solution: Health care organizations, hospitals and governmental agencies must be limited in the number or percentage of medical doctors in their direct employment, and have absolutely no authority to regulate medical doctors' patient-care decision making (it must be considered criminal activity if there is such interference). All medical doctors must otherwise maintain independent or group private practices. The private practice model must be mandatory for the majority of medical doctors. Of note, there appears to be a coordinated effort these days, by hospital organizations in collusion with government, to exterminate the concept of private practice. If the concept of private practice is not preserved, protected and brought back up to previous historic levels, then the American health care system is doomed to disaster. Additionally, all certificate of need regulations in every state must be abolished to allow free market forces to increase competition, increase innovation, increase choices and decrease prices.

8. "Health care" is "sick care" and "alternative" care is not health care. When you think about it, medical doctors do not necessarily focus on health – they focus on sickness and degeneration and injury. The idea is that allopathic medical doctors can find out what the medical problem is and then try to solve the problem or at least lessen or slow the impact of the problem. Medical doctors will be of better service to their patients to understand their potential role as protectors of health as well as healers. This will require greater clinical skill, greater wisdom, greater understanding of human nature, greater commitment to the practice of medicine as a calling or vocation, more hands-on involvement with patients and their lives, less personal devotion to research, greater independence from health care organizations and hospitals and academia and government, and a mindset that the focus needs to be on the patient and not on the doctor's microfame.

Obstacles to Patients Receiving Quality Care

The concept of "alternative" care usually connotes that a patient seeks care from some "provider" or "practitioner" or "clinician" that is not a true allopathic medical doctor. The underlying belief is that that there is some mystical healing force that is known only to such a practitioner, and that traditional true allopathic medical doctors don't know about this force. Typically, acupuncturists, massage therapists, chiropractors, reflexologists, herbalists, shamans, faith healers, homeopaths and naturopaths will fall under this category of alternative care practitioners. There is no mystical force other than the true and powerful concepts of placebo effect and hands-on care. Most of the time, when someone isn't feeling well, that person needs someone to touch them, to listen to them and to express a genuine care for them. That person needs to believe in the power of the care. It is for these reasons that "alternative" care can be useful for many people in many cases. The human body has a powerful ability to heal itself and when combined with the benefits of touch and of placebo effect, sometimes, that is all that is needed. However, to think that any of these alternative care treatments can be the preferable modalities to treat true medical or surgical maladies is beyond absurd – it is dangerous. Some of the alternative care modalities are clearly harmful and can make matters much worse. It is preferable that true allopathic medical doctors become well-versed in every type of alternative care concept and incorporate such modalities, while imposing appropriate limitations, into the overall care plan for every patient.

The placebo effect is often misunderstood. The placebo effect is a powerful healing phenomenon. It is real. It is not a fake treatment. It is not used exclusively for people who are "faking" their symptoms; it is most useful for people who have real symptoms. However, its beneficial effect is extremely limited in cases of more serious underlying medical or surgical maladies. In cases of more serious underlying medical or surgical maladies, appropriate pharmaceutical remedies or surgical interventions become absolutely necessary.

9. Low quality health care insurance. More and more patients are being shifted, sometimes against their will, to low quality health plans such as the federal Medicaid program and similar state run programs. These plans pay the doctors and facilities so little that it amounts to charity services. For a hypothetical example, if a doctor needs to charge $100 for a patient encounter, just to be able to stay in business and pay his expenses, and therefore needs $110 or more to actually get paid a token income for himself, the Medicaid-like program might pay something like $22.50 for the encounter. This means that the doctor not only didn't make money, but essentially had to give the patient $77.50 out of his own pocket in forced charity. Many doctors in the past would do this, but limit the number of Medicaid-type patients. This is nearly impossible for most doctors today. More patients are being put on Medicaid-type insurance policies only to find that no doctors are participating anymore. To make matters worse, any doctor that wants to participate in this entirely unfair, unsustainable, insane construct of an insurance program, will be put through excruciating scrutiny and have to fill out reams of paperwork and face unreasonable demands by unreasonable people within the system and face long wait times for approval. It is not worth the effort, because, when approved, it may be difficult to collect on any encounter due to a culture of sometimes denying doctors' payments for the silliest of reasons. The effort required to collect payment isn't worth the $22.50 that the doctor

will get. You would think that a system that calls upon doctors to be so charitable would make it easy for them and would be thankful to them, but it is quite the opposite.

Solution: No medical doctor or patient should participate in this type of program, and every governmental agency on a federal and state level must abandon this type of program as a dismal failure.

10. Increased access to health care. This statement may seem counterintuitive, but there is a medical doctor shortage right now. The prevailing (faulty) logic is that if patients have increased access to health care, then they will be healthier because diseases will be detected and treated before they progress too far to cause catastrophic consequences. However, some patients have such a low copay or no copay that they run to the doctor's office or emergency room for every little thing.   Due to the fear of malpractice lawsuits, doctors become obligated to do the million dollar work up every time. Not much thought and reason is put into the situation; just get tests and refer to specialists. So the health care system gets overwhelmed with patients that should not be patients at all, and often the true patients get lost in the system or care is needlessly delayed for them.

Chapter Five:

Obstacles to Medical Doctors Providing Quality Care

The following is a tip-of-the iceberg list of some of the things that prevent medical doctors from providing quality health care, rob them of time and money and needlessly add cost to the health care system:

1. Medicare: The system is gravely dysfunctional as it is, but on top of that there are annual radical changes monopolistically imposed on medical doctors. Doctors are fools for continuing to participate year after year in the Medicare system that year after year abuses them. There is a Stockholm syndrome going on here. At some point in the near future, every doctor needs to agree to disenrollment from Medicare at the same time. Until we are all willing to do this, the Medicare system will continue to abuse us, laugh at us, make fools of us and force us into taking bad care of our patients. When you consider the current issues regarding the Meaningful Use Program, the Pay for Performance Program, the Accountable Care Organization Program, the Medical Home Program, the Merit Based Incentive Payments System Program, the Alternative Payment Model Program, the Quality Payment Program, the Physician Quality Reports System Program, the Qualified Clinical Data Registry Program, the Delivery System Reform Program, the Medicare Payment Reform Program, the Medicare Access and CHIP Reauthorization Act, along with

whatever new ideological poison they'll be serving next year – it just becomes an annual festival of sadomasochism.

2. Medicaid: Any medical doctor who still participates in Medicaid is purely a fool or is otherwise bribed in some way, kind of like a prostitute for some organization. Any doctor who supports the Medicaid system is allowing such enrolled patients to be harmed – a clear violation of any doctor's oath.

3. The Patient Protection and Affordable Care Act [PPACA or ACA] and most other federal health care laws: These exist for the government by the government. We need to do away with all of them; for the people by the people.

4. Physician Payments Sunshine Act section of the ACA: A useless burdensome program whereby doctors need to go through a long drawn out cumbersome complicated unintuitive enrollment process and check into every month or so and have a chance to fight false information only a few weeks per year and little power to fight potentially defamatory information put there by pharmaceutical companies.

5. Health Insurance Portability and Accountability Act [HIPAA]: Most of this is needlessly complicated and often misunderstood and often unenforced. Some useful components are merely expressions of medical ethics and those concepts must be incorporated into the medical doctor's oath and incorporated into licensure requirements and not into federal law.

6. Malpractice issues: Malpractice systems in many states are set up to rob money from the health care system and give it to lawyers. As currently configured in some states, they serve no beneficial purpose to doctors or patients other than to put undue

burdens on both and raise costs to the health care system overall. An alternative system is immediately called for.

7. Electronic health records [EHRs] or sometimes known as electronic medical records [EMRs]: There is no proof that these provide any benefit to medical doctors or patients; however, there is some evidence to support the opposite. It puts people at high risk for identity theft, increases time demand for doctors taking them away from their patients and adds tremendous undue financial burden to the health care system. It was put in place by political hacks for the purpose of big business profit and enabling governmental control over the citizenry. There may be aspects of EHRs that are beneficial in some way to doctors and patients, but the adoption of such technology must be voluntary, optional and at the sole discretion of the treating medical doctor. If EHR features are of benefit to medical doctors, then adoption will increase naturally over time. However, currently, most EHRs inhibit the smooth functioning of a doctor's practice, are prohibitively costly (with no means of offset reimbursement) and interfere with the quality of patient care. The systems are being brutally forced upon doctors.

8. National Plan and Provider Enumeration System [NPPES] National Provider Identifier [NPI] number: I am not a person anymore: "They've given me a number, oh they've taken away my name" (from the 1966 song "Secret Agent Man"). Yet another bureaucratic agency that adds cost to the health care system, adds personnel and payroll to the federal government and serves no purpose. Medical doctors already have social security numbers and medical license numbers and board certification numbers.

9. Drug Enforcement Administration [DEA] number: A federal program that also gives a doctor a number and takes away his money, and is renewable every three years (for higher and higher fees with each renewal). Yet another bureaucratic agency that adds cost to the health care system, adds personnel and payroll to the federal government and serves no purpose. Medical doctors already have social security numbers and medical license numbers and board certification numbers.

10. Drug Control Registration: As if the federal DEA program is not enough, certain states have their own duplicated program to give doctors yet another number and to take away more money and to repeat the process every so many years. Yet another bureaucratic agency that adds cost to the health care system, adds personnel and payroll to the state government and serves no purpose. Medical doctors already have social security numbers and medical license numbers and board certification numbers.

11. State medical license: This is an appropriate but still needlessly burdensome credentialing process that could be streamlined for efficiency. This is typically administered by the board of medicine in each state. The board of medicine agency in each state is typically under-supported and under-utilized and could potentially consolidate many of the roles being senselessly duplicated in other state and federal agencies. Also, if a medical doctor has a license in one state, it means nothing in another state where the process would have to be started from scratch. It would be far more helpful to the health care system if once a medical doctor achieved licensure in one state, then there would be reciprocity in all other states with a fast simple application, one page with approval in one day. This would especially help

underserved areas to allow medical doctors to be more geographically fluid.

12. Board certification: As if going through medical school, passing all school tests, passing all national standardized tests, passing internship and tests, passing residency and tests, passing fellowship and tests and achieving the M.D. degree and a full medical license is not enough. In addition to that, medical doctors have to pay some self-appointed gang of hustler's exorbitant fees and take yet additional redundant unrelated certification exams just to be able to state the obvious: that the doctors went to medical school and trained in a certain path of medicine or surgery. This serves no purpose other than to cause doctors to spend more time away from patients and to take money away from doctors and give it to purposeless organizations which exist for the sole purpose of taking money away from doctors. No hospital or insurance carrier or credentialing body or medical doctor should participate with the board certification concept anymore. Furthermore, medical doctors should not be locked into a specific sub-field of the practice of medicine or surgery for their entire careers. It is counterproductive to the best service of their communities. Such a change would especially help underserved areas to allow medical doctors to be more specialty fluid. There must be mechanisms, such as mid-career apprenticeships, to allow easier transitions.

13. Maintenance of certification [MOC]: This is the same thing as board certification, but instead of a one-time thing, this entitles the hustlers to come after you time and time again to "maintain" the certification.

14. Sub-specialization fellowships and sub-specialization board certification: Here's a great idea that medical and surgical

training programs came up with: Let's delete certain aspects of training from the internship and residency training programs and then make the doctors come back for another year or three so we can get some more years of low-cost labor out of them and then train them in those things we should have trained them in during the residency, and let's call it a fellowship program. Then let's work in collusion with those hustlers, the board certification organizations, to add legitimacy to what we're doing, and they can create more ridiculous exams and charge more exorbitant fees and make more obscene profits and create board sub-specialization certification programs and create maintenance of sub-specialization certification programs.

15. Council for Affordable Quality Healthcare [CAQH]: This is an official, non-official, Washington D.C.-based nonprofit, non-governmental, centralized organization that many health insurance companies and other organizations and agencies turn to for credentialing information regarding individual medical doctors, and so doctors are forced to deal with this on a regular basis, essentially being harassed to keep up with this database program even though it is burdensome and provides no proven benefit to doctors or patients.

16. Credentialing and re-credentialing and re-credentialing — even when nothing changes: What is credentialing? It is filling out reams of paperwork or online database registries with every detail of your education and training and practice since high school, including college, medical school, internship, residency, fellowship, board certifications, maintenance of certifications, medical licensing, DEA certificates, state drug control registration certificates, employment history, letters of verification, letters of reference, letters of explanation of any irregularities,

testimonials, questionnaires, records of litigation, hospital affiliations, publications, malpractice insurance history, commercial insurance enrollment status, statements of personal health issues, etc., and, in most cases, paying a fee. Instead of doctors having to do credentialing and re-credentialing multiple times per year, year after year, with insurers, hospitals, CAQH, licensing or certification authorities, there must be one repository. The best potential repository is the states' boards of medicine. Each state board must collect and preserve the credentialing data, adding to the credentialing file only when there is a change, and sharing credentialing information, upon the doctor's authorization, with hospitals, insurers and others as needed. This will save medical doctors tremendous time each year.

17. Continuing medical education [CME]: Periodically burdensome, but absolutely necessary for medical doctors to keep up with lifelong education.

18. Practice management and scheduling software: Necessary these days to run a medical practice, but has added complexity to the more simple old fashion ways of running a medical office. A book can be written on this topic alone.

19. Physician hospital organizations [PHOs], or other phrases to that effect: These are organizations that medical doctors have joined, for an annual fee and with needlessly burdensome paperwork, with the intent of having collective representation as members of a hospital-affiliated community. The idea was that such an organization would protect the doctor's autonomy, against the machinations of the hospital administrators and health insurance companies, for the benefit of the patients in the community. These type of organizations still exist but rarely

represent the doctors for the benefit of the patients. They now represent the hospital for the benefit of negotiating higher payments to the hospital from patients and insurance carriers, even if it adds expense to the doctors. Such organizations have become venues whereby hospital administrators impose their will on doctors. Any doctor that does not comply may be banished, even if it reduces quality of patient care and increases costs.

20. Hospitals: Hospitals are necessary evils. It is often said that hospitals hate medical doctors and would get rid of all of them if they could. Hospitals want to own and control doctors and everything they do – and they typically make it nearly impossible for doctors to function effectively on quality of patient care. Hospitals make money only because doctors work there, and yet hospitals are paying doctors less and less over time. Administrators work much less than doctors, bring no money into the hospital, are being hired in increasing numbers, and yet make more money than doctors in many or most cases. I suggest that hospitals minimize their habit of directly employing medical doctors. I also suggest that hospitals incorporate medical doctors as administrators and avoid non-medical-doctor administrators.

21. Health care organizations: By this I mean large medical centers or hospital conglomerates. This is evil on steroids. Anything that is bad about a hospital is magnified to an extreme when all the hospitals combine into a local or regional monopoly health care organization. The patients and medical doctors are doomed in such cases. Costs go up, efficiency goes down, quality of care goes down, doctor excellence goes down, but profits for the conglomerate entity go up. Marketing propaganda for the conglomerate usually loses any connection to truth. Doctors may

be penalized or even driven out if they refer a patient outside of the organization, even if it is the right thing for the patient.

22. Health insurance companies: These days, health insurance companies are often just middlemen to siphon money out of the health care system so they can have lavish offices with ever growing highly paid staff to create ever increasingly complex transaction models. They even attempt to practice medicine without a license by dictating what medical doctors and patients can and cannot do. Additionally, they have been emboldened by being apparently exempt from anti-trust or anti-collusion regulations and so some of them engage in industry-coordinated price-fixing against patients and doctors. It is ironic that a doctor must post a specific fee schedule, with an immutable price per CPT code, which must be the same for all patients and all insurance companies; however, insurance companies can have multiple fee schedules and varying prices per CPT code depending on the doctor or hospital. Two doctors practicing in the same building, practicing the same specialty, seeing the same patient for the same diagnosis, billing the same CPT code, can be paid two different amounts by the same insurance company, even if each doctor's fee for that CPT code is the same. Health insurance companies must be subject to anti-trust and anti-collusion regulations. Health insurance companies must abandon the concept of doctors "in network" and have one fee structure for all doctors even across state lines (for when patients travel). It can be more like car insurance. When an accident happens, the insurance company doesn't prevent you from going to the body shop of your choice, even if out of state, it just pays for the work to get done.

23. Prior authorizations: This is the insane but lawful (shouldn't be) concept whereby a person, sometimes without even a high school diploma, working at a call center for a health insurance company, can dictate what test a medical doctor can or cannot order for a patient. Imagine that, the medical doctor, with all his training and experience, after interviewing and examining the patient, being duly licensed and having the appropriate authority and experience, orders a test and a random person on the other end of the phone can say no and even go so far as to dictate what alternative (cheaper) test the doctor should order. The doctor and his staff can put up a long battle involving phone calls and paperwork and time delay to eventually get the correct test approved, but the doctor will not be compensated for this work in any way.

24. Formulary, either at the hospital or related to Medicare or Medicaid or related to a commercial health insurance company policy: Similar to the prior authorization process, if a medical doctor believes that a certain prescription is necessary for a patient, the hospital administrator policy or the governmental or commercial insurance company policy may deny it because it is not allowed in their formulary or because there is a policy which requires the patient to "fail" at least two cheaper alternative prescriptions first. However, the patient may suffer and the doctor will still be held accountable for the poor outcome, and may even be sued for malpractice. The doctor and his staff can put up a long battle involving phone calls and paperwork and time delay to eventually get the correct medication approved, but the doctor will not be compensated for this work in any way.

25. Increased access: It was thought that patients do not have enough easy access to medical doctors. Today the opposite is

true in many regions. Today a patient can decide to go to a doctor or a hospital at any time, even every day if he wants. This is crowding the emergency rooms, urgent care centers, clinics and offices with hypochondriacs and delaying access for those who really need it. To be fair, doctors need to learn better skills at treating hypochondriacs.

26. Perpetually reducing income: Year after year for the past ten to fifteen years, medical doctors' effective take home income, especially when adjusting for inflation, has been going down. I estimate that doctors have to see twice as many patients today as they did ten years ago just to make the same take home pay. It gets worse: The general public has had the long-held misconception that medical doctors are "rich" and that money is just flowing like Niagara Falls into every medical doctor's practice. Because of this misconception, every conceivable governmental and nongovernmental organization has put an annually ever increasing parasitic mandatory financial bite into doctors' practices. They rationalize: "They make so much money, we'll just take a little and they won't know the difference." However, after the one thousandth entity latches on, the doctor's practice is driven to desperate financial acts or otherwise dies.

27. Perpetually increasing costs: The amount of money that is paid to a medical doctor's office is not the doctor's income. All of the office expenses, practice fees, malpractice insurance premiums, equipment costs, medical supplies costs, taxes, utilities, rent, payroll and other overhead is deducted first and then the doctor gets what is left over (at some times of the year, there is nothing left over). Payments per case to doctors are less each year, but overhead is more. This is unsustainable.

28. Built in obsolescence of technology: As one of many examples, when Windows XP went to Windows 7 and all the electronic health records software and business practice software and even hardware needed to be upgraded for compatibility, it caused a serious behind the scenes crash of the entire health care industry in many regions throughout the country. So many people could not adapt to the forced changes and many doctors and practice managers went into early retirement. Many doctor's offices and some hospitals just did not upgrade, and so faced dysfunctionality and increased security risks. At the same time certain biomedical technology equipment needed to be upgraded such as imaging hardware, electrodiagnostic equipment and neurophysiological testing equipment. I could list many such examples. This kind of thing keeps happening with hardware, software and biomedical technology. It may be fun and exciting for the general citizen to buy a new smart phone every 18 months, and it may be a highly desirable source of renewable profits for technology and computer companies; however, a doctor's office runs best if it can keep its technology stable for at least 20 or 30 years. Such upgrades and advances do not necessarily enhance medical practices, more often they interfere with medical practices. The new features are often useless to doctors. An electroencephalogram machine from 20 years ago might work just as well as one from today, in some cases, it might work better. To be forced to get a new machine at a great cost when the doctor still hasn't paid off the old one, just because the new one can communicate with a new EHR module through the internet that the doctor doesn't even use, and is imposed because a lobbyist convinced a politician legislator that it was a great idea, has become intolerable and unsustainable.

29. Risk to medical doctor's own health or life from patients' contagious illnesses.

30. Risk to medical doctor's own health or life from patient violent attacks, especially regarding attempts to manipulate the doctor concerning disability claims, workers compensation claims and opioid medication prescriptions. Sometimes violence against doctors is a result of mental illness in their patient.

31. Medical doctors are human and have family responsibilities and personal tragedies.

32. Algorithms and guidelines and protocols: In most cases created and imposed (by virtue of penalty) by people and committees and organizations and agencies that do not involve medical doctors.   In most cases, inappropriate or at best inadequate to deal with any unique individual patient.

33. Burdens of ever increasing senseless complexities of small business regulations.

34. Academic bias: Many medical doctors are brainwashed into (mistakenly) believing that they must be on a professorship tract affiliated with a medical school in order to achieve credibility as a medical doctor. This creates a terrible conflict of interest for many reasons. As one example, the doctor will be forced to see a patient encounter not as an opportunity to help the patient, but as an opportunity to enroll a test subject into the research project currently going on in their academic department. They should disclose this conflict of interest, and patients would be best served to avoid such doctors.

35. Publications: Many medical doctors, especially academic doctors and researcher doctors, are pressured to spend the bulk

of their time working on their next publication and hence they see patient care as a distraction from their primary purpose which is to achieve fame and influence in the medical community.

36.   Tiers: Some health insurance organizations have implemented a "Tier" structure to rate medical doctors who participate in their networks and policies.   It is a three tier structure with the insurance organization implying that tier one equates to best quality and that tier three equates to lowest quality.   What they don't tell you is that they define highest quality as the doctor that spends the least money on his patients. If I see my patient but do not order any test or prescribe any medication or perform any surgery, then I will be tier one – even if the patient seriously needs testing or medication or surgery.   No doctor and no patient should pay any attention to the tier concept – or else seek out tier two and three doctors and avoid tier one doctors.   (Watch what will happen now, the insurance companies will reverse the tiers and so the cheap lazy doctors will become tier three.)

37.   A medical doctor's own health insurance and that which he provides for his staff – especially considering the ever increasing costs involved.

38.   Insurance claims processing, collections and denials: Medicare and commercial insurance companies may pay medical doctors less and less each year, and as if that wasn't bad enough, sometimes Medicare and the commercial insurance companies just won't pay.   They may provide no legitimate reason (in the doctor's opinion).   The doctors then have to go through incredible efforts or even legal action just to get paid.   This can sometimes put a practice out of business.   Medicare and commercial insurance companies pay a fraction of what doctors bill or of what

doctors need to sustain their practices financially. Doctors often then turn to alternative forms of revenue which then distract doctors away from patient care. It is increasingly common for doctors to leave clinical practice to go to work for a pharmaceutical company or a biomedical technology company or a law firm or even Wall Street just to earn a salary commensurate with his level of training and expertise.

39. Alarmingly increasing rates of medical doctor burnout and suicide.

40. International Statistical Classification of Diseases and Related Health Problems [ICD] codes; currently at ICD-10: Medical doctors can't give you a diagnosis when submitting an invoice to your health care insurance company; they have to use an ICD code, these codes change every so many years and serve no purpose to the doctor or the patient. With each new iteration they become less useful, more complicated and waste more of the doctors' time. They must be abolished or simplified, or at least made voluntary and not mandatory. The ICD system is maintained by the World Health Organization [WHO] and it represents the American health care system (inappropriately) complying with attempts at globalist integration of health care management.

41. Current Procedural Terminology [CPT] codes: This is like ICD, except it codes for what the medical doctor did during the encounter. The doctor can't just say I examined the patient, diagnosed and prescribed. He can't just say I did spine surgery. He has to use a specific code. These codes may change every year and they serve no purpose to the doctor or the patient. They waste the doctors' time. They must be abolished or simplified, or at least made voluntary and not mandatory. The CPT system is

proprietary and is maintained by the American Medical Association [AMA]. It has been perpetually adopted by the Medicare system and commercial insurers (for profit to the AMA), and so this sets up a potential conflict of interest by the AMA against the doctors they purport to represent.

42. Referrals: This is a concept whereby a primary care medical doctor physician formally "refers" a patient to a specialist medical doctor. Some insurance companies and some health care organizations have strict prohibitions against referrals. In other words, primary care doctors are no longer allowed to refer their patients to the best specialist for the patient's needs. The insurance company may not pay for certain specialists because they are not affiliated with that insurance company. This is particularly common with certain restrictive employer-sponsored plans. In other cases, the primary care physician may be financially penalized by his affiliated health care organization if he refers "outside" the system, even if it best for the patient. In no case must a patient's freedom to seek the most appropriate specialist medical doctor be obstructed; such behavior must be made unlawful.

43. Prohibition against unionizing or collective bargaining or striking: All other American humans can do this. I guess the government does not consider medical doctors human. In many ways, medical doctors seem to be denied the Equal Protection Clause of the Fourteenth Amendment of the United States Constitution and denied the Due Process Clause of the Fifth Amendment of the United States Constitution.

44. Medical doctors may be annually victimized by some insurance companies which are apparently allowed to engage in collusion and price fixing against medical doctors because some

health care insurance companies seem to be exempt from such collusion and antitrust regulations.

45. Unfavorable tax considerations and AMT: Many private practice doctors become inappropriately subjected to the alternative minimum tax [AMT] by the IRS, and hence lose many personal deductions, because their gross business income is inappropriately recognized by the IRS as their gross personal income, instead of analyzing their net business income after business expenses as gross personal income.

46. Student loan debt: Many medical doctors, especially those just starting out at this time may be facing up to $500,000.00 in student loan debt and accruing interest after the loan deferral period. Add to that business practice start-up costs, home mortgage, family expenses, decreasing reimbursements, and many doctors live a life of near poverty through residency and early years of practice. Announcement: medical doctors are not "rich" anymore – they haven't been for decades and likely never will be again. Doctors are white collar professionals on a blue collar income.

49. Medical doctors almost never get paid for teaching, but are almost always required to teach. Often, the teaching facility then benefits from the clinical work the medical doctor does at the teaching facility.

50. Like most professionals today, doctors are flooded with emails: Typically, medical doctors will receive hundreds per day, many of an urgent or serious or time-sensitive nature. Medical doctors often must maintain multiple email accounts in addition to being forced to maintain other multiple alternative forms of electronic communication imposed by hospitals or EHRs.

Obstacles to Medical Doctors Providing Quality Care

Chapter summary: Over the years, medical doctors have entirely lost any semblance of control over their own profession. Many well-intentioned features, requiring additional costs and additional time commitments, have been imposed on doctors' practices by well-meaning people in positions of influence and control. Each feature may be considered logical and reasonable in isolation, but when they are all added up, they become paralyzing. There is no more time for doctors to see patients. There is no more money to take away from doctors.

When you have 500 different committees of people at 500 different agencies or organizations all imposing this logic, year after year, each believing they're the only one making just a little change to the doctor's practice, then we wind up where we are now: in a nasty web of bureaucratic and financial strangulation that is killing the sanctity of the doctor-patient relationship and driving doctors out of business.

Chapter Six:

Lawyers and Health Care

1. It is often joked that if you were stranded on a deserted island, who would you rather have with you a doctor or a lawyer? Of course, everybody says a doctor. This is sometimes extrapolated to explain how lawyers are not necessary. However, the United States of America is not a deserted island, and our society needs lawyers because they provide the necessary force that holds our civilization in balance. Without them, we would fall apart into anarchy or else coalesce into fascism. However, their place in the American health care system needs to be limited.

2. The legal profession's intrusion on American culture has become extreme, and our country is no longer a capitalistic republic, but instead has become what I call a legalopoly. I define legalopoly as the condition whereby society is monopolized by lawyers and litigation. Nearly all aspects of our American lives have been reconfigured to appease lawyers' views of the world. Nearly all aspects of our American lives are now preconfigured for the potential of future litigation. Real people shouldn't have to live this way – it's not healthy for the mind or body. Also, laws don't seem to apply to lawyers and legislators; they will always know how to get around them or else make themselves exempt. Medical doctors are now forced to write every patient-encounter note in a format that prepares the note for litigation, even if that format interferes with the efficacy and efficiency of patient care. Medical doctors now spend too much time preparing such legal

documents after every patient encounter; this distracts from quality of patient care.

As a curious consideration: A typical medical doctor may spend one hour with a patient and spend an additional 30 minutes researching and drafting a three page detailed document with potential legal ramifications, which could endure for a decade or more, that could leave that doctor in a position to spend three to five years in intensive litigation and potentially lose his life's savings, and he will be paid $128.00 for this document and this risk. If you asked a lawyer to do something similar, first of all, he wouldn't, second of all, if he did, he would get paid thousands of dollars and make sure he had no liability after the ink was dry.

3. Malpractice lawsuits, as currently configured in some states, exist primarily for the profit of trial lawyers and the legal profession. Legislators and judges are often complicit in this severe conflict of interest. Most malpractice cases are frivolous and baseless, but most of the cases are not dismissed because the judges that decide the cases might have been trial lawyers or might want to work for a trial law firm in the future, and they believe that any case is a good case because it keeps the business and the money flowing. Most of the money, in many of the cases, goes to the lawyers, not to the patient claimants. The lawyers will get money for their time, fees and expenses, and then get an additional sizeable percentage of the settlement or award. I suspect there are cases where ultimately all of the money goes to the lawyer and the patient winds up with nothing.

4. In malpractice cases, some lawyers are not interested in truth and justice, they are interested in winning and money. They may do anything and everything to destroy the doctor or hospital,

even if it is untrue, unethical and even unlawful (as long as they can get away with it). It is often said that decades or even centuries of malpractice litigation has contributed no significant improvement to health care or significant positive changes to medical care practices. However, it has caused substantial increase in health care costs due to ever increasing malpractice insurance premiums and due to the astronomically pervasive practice of defensive medicine.

Defensive medicine is loosely defined as a doctor ordering additional tests and procedures and consults and documentation just in case a lawyer might sue, but not because the patient needs such things.

Malpractice litigation has caused some rural or urban underserved areas to suffer the loss of certain specialists who refuse to practice knowing that the risk of undue litigation is high. Malpractice litigation has also caused pharmaceutical companies to discontinue certain drugs and vaccines, which may have been helpful or even lifesaving to thousands of people, due to the high risk of undue litigation. Doctors have become less interested in helping people with complicated or difficult medical issues because the outcome will be poor. The lawyers will sue due to the poor outcome, not due to anything the doctor did. Sometimes lawyers adopt the cavalier attitude: "It's no big deal, we just take the money from the malpractice insurance company, not the doctor..." But they will permanently destroy the doctor's reputation, even if the doctor ultimately wins the case. They also don't seem to consider the time and mental energy they drain from the doctor (as well as the patient claimants) during the years of litigation – this impairs the doctor's ability to take care of patients.

5. Solution: Replace the malpractice system with a no fault insurance program for patients. There are numerous potential ways of funding the program. The most logical way to fund it would be an annual fee extracted from doctors and hospitals. The program could be managed by the state. Lawyers would not be needed. The patient would fill out a simple claim, a panel made up of doctor representatives and patient representatives could decide the claims, and there would be certain time limits and award limits as per the state. This program could be administered through the states' boards of medicine.

With this kind of system in place, doctors could use their own clinical judgment regarding ordering of tests and treatments and even use their own judgment in how they speak to patients. Doctors of the past were seen as the anchors of strength and hope. The doctor was there to tell you it was going to be alright. He was there to instill confidence because having confidence that you will heal can have a healing effect. Doctors of today, trained under the current mindset of our legalopoly, are obligated to make you aware of every possible bad outcome, real or imagined, rare or common, introduce confusion, add doubt and cause insecurity. The loss of confidence can severely disrupt healing.

6. Of course this proposed program would not apply if the doctor engaged in criminal or fraudulent activity with respect to a patient.

7. The current American system of civil litigation is cruel and unfair. In criminal cases, the accused is innocent until proven guilty beyond reasonable doubt. However, in civil cases, the accused is guilty until he can prove he is not guilty beyond reasonable doubt. The person (or law firm) with the most money wins. When you are found to be not guilty, after you have spent

years of your life fighting and have consumed your life savings, you have no recourse to get your money back. Anybody can accuse anybody of anything in a lawsuit, even if it is a lie. This is psychologically and financially damaging to our society – very unhealthy. People who are facing civil litigation, especially when it is inappropriate (as in many cases), almost always develop medical problems requiring medical care. This dysfunctional system is a significant cause of morbidity in America. It can lead to chronic sleep disturbance, psychological or psychiatric issues, anxiety, depression, fainting, seizures, chronic gastrointestinal issues, heart attacks, strokes, and more.

8. The current system of civil litigation needs to be abandoned and replaced by a system that protects the innocence of the accused until proven, beyond reasonable doubt, guilty. The new system must bar lawyers from taking cases on contingency fees. All players need to have something at risk, it can't be seen as a lottery ticket. The new system must require payment of legal fees and expenses and payment for lost time to the accused if the accuser does not win, including coverage of medical care costs if a medical issue arose due to the litigation.

9. This new system must be mandated by federal and state legislation, but many legislators are lawyers, and many are trial lawyers, so there is a substantial disincentive. All lawyers must recuse themselves from voting, if such legislation comes up for a vote, due to the obvious conflict of interest.

10. It may be reasonable to create a new legal system whereby no person ever pays a lawyer directly. It will be done through insurance policies, and the insurers can dictate to the lawyers what the lawyers can charge and collect from their clients, and how much of a copay the clients will owe the lawyers. All citizens

will be required to have legal insurance, and all lawyers will be obligated to operate under this system. There can be federal government programs like Legalcare for the elderly and Legalaid for the poor. This would solve the serious acute legal system crisis that exists in America today. The federal government can then mandate that all lawyers use one particular computer system to enter all their case data, viewable by all lawyers and all government agents. The clients must have access to this online database and must be able to communicate with their lawyers through the database email system free of charge for any and all email communication. The government and insurance companies can regulate what lawyers must include in their notes. The government can disallow any tax write offs when lawyers' fees or expenses aren't covered by the client or the client's insurance. The government and insurance companies can require lawyers to follow a coding system which identifies the nature of the legal case (civil fraud is code 12.074, criminal larceny is code 14.027, etc.) – and if the coding is wrong, then the lawyers cannot get paid. The government and insurance companies can require lawyers to follow a coding system which identifies the nature of the legal procedure (deposition is code F-56, court appearance is code G-92, etc.) – and if the coding is wrong, then the lawyers cannot get paid.

It is abusive how lawyer-politicians have thought up this kind of system for medical doctors' payments, while they would never impose it on themselves. It was through pure gullibility and passiveness that doctors have let this happen. It is self-destructive and masochistic that doctors continue to participate.

Chapter Seven:

The Right to Freedom of Health Care

1. With the primary focus on doctors and patients, it is proposed that a new amendment be added to the United States Constitution. The primary purpose is to consider freedom of health care as a right for all citizens of the United States of America.

2. I will remind readers that, in America, when you are given a right to something, that does NOT mean that the government must provide it for you; it DOES mean that you are entitled to pursue this free from governmental interference. If the government provides something for you then that is considered an entitlement.

3. A secondary purpose of this proposed new amendment is to prevent the encroachment of governmental influence, whether it be federal or state or regional or local or municipal, into the power and responsibility of diagnosis and treatment decisions which must be protected under the exclusive control and jurisdiction of true allopathic medical doctors.

4. Governmental bodies, with the excuse of cost containment or "quality" oversight or other propagandish reasons, have desired to control the American health care system and medical doctors. The true motives have been multifactorial and variable over time, but always against the best interest of doctors and patients.

5. All health care is local. All health care is individual. Diagnostic and treatment standards work best when they are developed and perpetually updated locally by clinical allopathic medical doctors based on the combination of education, training, experience, wisdom, ethics, feedback, review, current science, available technology and peer collaboration, all custom-applied to the individual patient.

6. It makes no sense that any governmental body – being completely detached and distant to the patient – should have any say in the doctor-patient relationship. Every governmental body is composed of people who have little or no medical training or clinical medical experience, and have no right or authority to practice medicine as individuals or as organizational bodies, and yet that is the effect of what has been happening in America: organizations practicing medicine without due authority.

7. Governmental officials, governmental agencies, third party insurance payers, lawyers, judges, courts, employers, business entities, hospitals, health care organizations, physicians' organizations, professional organizations, international organizations, pharmacies, pharmaceutical companies, biomedical technology companies and even academic medical institutions all have extreme biases and conflicts of interest which are usually against the best interest of medical doctors and patients.

8. Governmental agencies may hire what they perceive as "experts" in the field of health care such as academic medical doctors, hospital administrators, insurance company executives, delegates from professional medical associations, financial budgeteers, legal scholars and health care related lobbyists as consultants to develop diagnostic and treatment algorithms or

guidelines or protocols, inclusion criteria, exclusion criteria, threshold data, prior authorization rules and so on. This imposes central regulation on the doctor-patient relationship – based on the faulty assumption that only these "smart" people can see the big picture and know what is best for all parties involved. Clearly, these notions and methodologies are severely flawed.

9. The clinical allopathic medical doctor, practicing within the constraints of that individual's training, experience, expertise, credentialing, culture and geographic location, is the single best authority to evaluate a patient, make a diagnosis and implement a treatment.

10. I hereby submit the following proposal to the U.S. House of Representatives and to the U.S. Senate with the hope that they will take whatever action necessary to establish this as the next (28th) amendment to the United States Constitution. The following proposed amendment is intended to preserve independence for the patient and for the doctor against the government, against lawyers and against big business. We can call it the Right to Freedom of Health Care.

Section 1: The rights of the citizens of the United States, who are 18 years or older, to privately engage health care services from duly licensed medical doctors, whether through direct compensation or through any third party compensation, on their own behalf or on behalf of any minor under their guardianship, shall not be denied or abridged by the United States or by any state for any reason at any time.

Section 2: The right of an appropriately trained and licensed medical doctor to privately engage in providing commensurate health care services to citizens of the United States shall not be denied or abridged by the United States or by any state for any reason at any time, and shall never be made contingent upon direct employment by the United States or any state, and shall never be made contingent upon compulsory participation in any United-States-funded or any state-funded insurance program or direct-pay program, and shall never be made contingent upon compliance with any United-States-imposed or any state-imposed diagnostic or treatment criteria, algorithm, guideline or protocol, and shall never be allowed to be made contingent upon compliance with any third-party-payer-imposed diagnostic or treatment criteria, algorithm, guideline or protocol. Additionally, the action of any appropriately trained and licensed medical doctor to engage in providing commensurate health care services to citizens of the United States shall never be forced by the United States or any state for any reason at any time in any way.

Section 3: Every citizen of the United States must procure protection against errors, omissions or mistakes made by duly licensed medical doctors practicing lawfully in the United States or its territories in the form of no-fault mishap health care insurance coverage. The funding of such insurance may be through payroll tax or fees imposed on medical doctors or such insurance may be purchased privately by any citizen. The determination of compensation to any patient claimant related to claims against such insurance coverage must be expeditiously administered under the direction of a body composed equally of medical doctors and patient representative overseers unrelated to the entity providing the insurance coverage and unrelated to any persons involved in the claim. Any compensation granted to a patient claimant, due as a result of any successful claim under this section, must be distributed urgently and must be one hundred percent retained by the patient claimant and no amount shall be due to, or shared with, any third party, even an attorney or advocate.

Section 4: The right of appropriately trained and licensed medical doctors to diagnose, treat and otherwise practice within the scope of their training, licensure and experience shall be immune against civil lawsuits as brought by any citizen or patient, regardless of the outcome of any doctor-patient interaction. This section does not provide immunity to, or protection against, issues relating to the fraudulent practice of health care or any criminal activity.

Section 5: The Congress shall have power to enforce this amendment by appropriate legislation.

Chapter Eight:

Patient Protection and Affordable Care Act

1. The Patient Protection and Affordable Care Act [PPACA or ACA] was passed by the federal government and made into law in the year 2010. It was marketed as having an intent to protect patients and improve affordability of health care insurance and of health care services. It achieved the opposite of protecting patients, and it has increased the costs of health care. Like everything else that comes from Washington D.C. politicians, it has an appealing name but it does the opposite of what it says. This Act represents a compilation of stream of consciousness ideological machinations collected into a manual developed by lobbyists and political party operatives working together to gain control over the American health care system, neuter the medical profession, invade the privacy of citizens and unconstitutionally entitle the federal government to supersede states' rights.

2. The ACA is a long and complicated mish mosh of legislation that was passed in a draft format because of power struggles and fighting between political parties. This Act is not a clear and concise legislative product that was thoughtfully created by medical doctors and patients and legislators working together for the betterment of the country's health care system.

3. The Democrats cared about winning the fight, no matter what. Some of their party leaders were proud of themselves for finding unethical immoral methods to force the draft-law through. They

did not care about patients or doctors or American civilization. They cared about their pride and they were loyal to their party – they were traitors to their country. The Republicans cared about winning the fight. Some of their party leaders were focused on blocking, rather than recognizing their weak position and trying to mitigate the damage that this law would cause. They did not care about patients or doctors or American civilization. They cared about their pride and they were loyal to their party – they were traitors to their country. Democrats and Republicans in the Senate and in the House of Representatives, all of them at that moment in American history, were abject failures, betrayed their oaths of office and betrayed their president who has, in years since, been left trying to defend their indefensible acts of betrayal to the American people.

I am no Constitutional scholar or legal historian; however, I do know that the separation of powers means that the executive branch works in opposition to the other two branches, and the legislative branch (Senate and House) works in opposition to the other two branches, and the judicial branch works in opposition to the other two branches. In this way there are checks and balances to prevent tyranny. We now have tyranny in America perpetrated by the government because of the two party system. The government is no longer managed by the checks and balances of branches of government, it is run by whichever political party has most control over the branches.

Our founding fathers wisely never intended for there to be political parties and never intended for people to be career politicians. People would go to Washington part time, be paid little, be there a limited time, represent the best interests of the people from their communities, then go back home, get back to work in the private sector and let the next person have a turn. Having openly declared political parties is better than having secretive political parties. There is not much we can do about it – except to encourage senators and congressman to represent their constituents and represent the legislative branch, and to absolutely avoid representing their political party due to the blatant and harmful conflict of interest.

The presidency is intended to be a powerful leadership position. You may not like the direction a particular president takes the country, but he does have the authority to do so. Due to term limits and various checks and balances and laws, the direction can be limited and then changed again by the next president.

The judicial branch, especially considering the U.S. Supreme Court, is often driven by political ties and not by the pursuit of truth and justice. Decisions are sometimes made based on political ideologies and political affiliations – not based on law, not based on the Constitution and not based on what is right. The following are suggested solutions: Require that every Supreme Court decision must be 100% unanimous rather than majority – and the justices cannot come out of their chambers until they reach a unanimous decision. Require that the justices must not all be lawyers, and must all demonstrate continual competency in adhering to the United States Constitution. Require each to pass a periodic certification test demonstrating an understanding of the Constitution. Require term limits. Some of them get senile or demented in office or are influenced by substance abuse. Require them to go through random screening for illicit drugs and alcohol toxicity – and removed if caught with such substances in their bodies. Require that ten justices form the body of the U.S.

Supreme Court, a limit of five chosen by each major party, and that no case can be brought before the court unless all ten are present.

Since lobbyists and special interest groups control the majority of senators and congressman, perhaps there should be a third division of the legislative branch of the federal government. Leave the U.S. Senate to represent the states' interests. Leave the U.S. House of Representatives to represent the states' citizenry, but create the "U.S. House of Commerce" to represent businesses and special interests groups. This tricameral approach would provide for improved transparency and better representation for all.

I see all politicians as avatars for controlling oligarchs (I don't know who the oligarchs are, but I'm sure they're there). The oligarchs, through surreptitious financial manipulations, install the politicians in their respective offices, in many cases against the will of the people. The oligarchs, sometimes in collusion with corporate or international allegiances, design and plan the direction of domestic and foreign policies and then pull the strings of their avatar politicians (senators, congressman, presidents, judges, etc.) to impose their will. Such is the current influence over health care policy in America today.

4. It is tremendously unfortunate that the components of the ACA law that have received national attention and have been brought to litigation are the most trivial aspects of the law. Regarding the doctor-patient relationship, it doesn't matter if health insurance companies are being forced to keep children on their parent's policies until the age of 26 and it doesn't matter if all citizens are required to obtain health insurance policies otherwise face a tax or a penalty. Those are financial matters

affecting individuals and health insurance companies, and have caused increases of health care costs, but have otherwise not impacted patient care quality.

5. The more sinister components embedded in the ACA empower the federal government to take control over nearly every aspect of the doctor-patient relationship and indirectly enable the federal government to supersede the states' rights to regulate medical doctors. This sinister authority makes up the bulk of the ACA. It surprises me that not much has been reported about this because this is where the real harm to the American people will come from. Perhaps since many of these components are phased in slowly over many years and since the impact won't be noticed for years after that, then nobody is focusing on it now – this represents a premeditated, intentional, insidious, fundamentally transformational destruction of our once great American health care system.

6. The language of the ACA is purposefully vague so that the meaning can be manipulated by lawyers and politicians and judges and businesses to extract almost any kind of influence and control over medical doctors and patients eventually in the future.

7. See Chapter Nine in this book about section 6002 of the ACA, and how it inappropriately controls and harms doctors and causes increase of health care costs.

8. See Chapter Fifteen in this book about the concept of electronic health records [EHRs], and how it inappropriately controls and harms doctors and patients.

9. The propaganda that was used to enable the ACA was the creation of the myth that the American health care system was in

crisis, and the federal government needed to step in and fix it. It was not in crisis then, but it is in crisis now. In order to fix it we need the federal government to step out of it. The health care system had aspects that were dysfunctional and the two most dysfunctional aspects of the health care system, the need for proper malpractice reform and the need to convert Medicare back to just an insurance plan, were not addressed at all.

10. Although there are a few beneficial aspects of the ACA, those are miniscule compared to the tsunami of disastrous aspects and so the only solution is complete repeal. If legislators, working with true clinical allopathic medical doctors and working with patients, desire to subsequently draft simple legislation to address important issues one at a time, then that might be appropriate. It is a manipulative myth that we needed then, or need now, some overarching mega health care law to govern medical doctors and patients and insurance companies and pharmaceutical companies.

Chapter Nine:

The Physician Payments Sunshine Act

1. This is more precisely known as section 6002 of the Patient Protection and Affordable Care Act [ACA]. It is managed through a subsection of the Center for Medicare and Medicaid Services [CMS] known as the Open Payments Program based on its "final rule." It is a bureaucratic nightmare that increases the cost of health care, puts undue unfair burden on medical doctors' time, puts undue and unfair burden on the pharmaceutical industry, has harmed many local economies, has diminished sources of medical doctors' supplemental income, has caused pharmaceutical company employees to face unemployment, and was designed and implemented with no evidence that it would be of any benefit to anyone. I choose this topic to explore in greater detail as just one example among thousands of similar topics that destructively intrude on the medical profession. Extrapolate this analysis to the other thousands of topics, most of which are far more complex and intrusive, and you will begin to understand the dangerous absurdity of it all.

2. The thought behind the program is based on woefully outdated issues. Decades ago, in the United States, pharmaceutical companies used to shower certain doctors and their families with money and gifts such as family trips to the Caribbean, new cars, lavish meals at fine restaurants, etc. In return, the doctors would be spokesmen to promote the branded products of the company. The doctor's endorsement would add credibility to the product. I am not aware of any situation whereby the doctor would

prescribe, or encourage prescribing, the product if it wasn't appropriate for the patient. Every doctor would still be responsible for, and interested in, the outcome of the patient. However, if prescribing occurs purely as quid-pro-quo for financial gain, that has always been considered criminal activity. Doctors were not likely to promote a product that was harmful, and besides, every product would have already passed FDA approval. However, this issue became one of the APPEARANCE of conflict of interest. Decades ago, this behavior was discontinued by self-policing; by both the pharmaceutical industry and the professional medical community. There were also some states that created legislation to deal with this. By the year 2010, the potential problems had long since been resolved, with doctors receiving only modest compensation, no lavish gifts, no spouses or family allowed to be involved, and the requirement for full disclosure.

3. Politicians may take thousands and millions of dollars from special interests and lobbyists during their campaigns and while in office, but they insist that there is no chance for conflict of interest or influence (when there clearly is). However, they will create complicated laws to oversee, prevent and punish medical doctors if they so much as accept a branded pen or a sandwich from a pharmaceutical company due to the potential for conflict of interest (when there clearly isn't).

4. The way the law works is that if a pharmaceutical company or one of its representatives provides something of financial value (such as a speaking fee, a meal, a medical book, etc.), then the company needs to report all of the details of that transaction, and of every transaction, to the federal government. If it is not reported within a certain timeframe, or if it is incorrectly

reported, there will be substantial financial penalties to the company. The company has the responsibility to go through a complicated sign up process to register an account with the federal government, and has to continually maintain the account for every doctor and hospital it does business with, as well as hire a legal team to oversee it. This adds a tremendous unnecessary burden to the pharmaceutical industry and ultimately adds costs to the health care system. Most importantly, this does not improve health care quality for patients.

5. Medical doctors need to go through a lengthy, complicated and needlessly burdensome process to create and maintain and frequently check an account with the federal government (if they don't check in within every 60 day interval they have to start the lengthy burdensome process all over again). Only once per year, for only a few weeks window of opportunity, medical doctors can log in and review what the pharmaceutical companies have published about them regarding financial transactions, and have a chance to dispute. Much, if not most, of what is put there by some pharmaceutical companies is false.

6. Due to the heavy financial penalties put on the pharmaceutical companies, they tend to err on the side of over-reporting rather than risk facing a penalty. Conflicts arise when, for example, a company sales representative's job or salary or bonus depends on meeting with as many medical doctors as possible. So the rep over-reports which doctors he met with and which doctors he left promotional material with. It looks good for the rep and the rep gets to keep his job another year, or gets a bonus. Reps have gotten creative as many doctors no longer let them in their offices, and so the reps will leave "educational material" or even things like donuts with the receptionists, and claim credit for

"meeting with the doctor." The doctor may never even know about the educational material which was thrown in the trash, or the donuts which were eaten by the staff.

I had an incident last year: the rep reported that she brought a luncheon to my office for me and my staff, and that she provided abundant educational material and that she gave a promotional presentation to my whole office. I could easily prove that I was out of the state on that date, and our office was closed. However, it took me weeks of back and forth emails and phone calls and ultimately threats of litigation to have the false information removed from my record. I don't get paid for such time wasted, and patients don't get taken care of when I waste my time dealing with things like that.

7. The CMS Open Payments Program website is there to allow reporting transactions and filing of disputes, but will not become arbiter of the disputes. Furthermore, in every case, the doctor is considered guilty unless he can convince or sue the reporting pharmaceutical company, and succeed at that in a very short window of time each year (weeks). The doctors have to continually monitor the data, even if they have no involvement with pharmaceutical companies. The pharmaceutical companies face no penalties within this system for false reporting of this nature. This further takes doctors away from patient care and adds to the ever growing burden which is leading most doctors to early burnout.

8. The irony is that there is nothing wrong with doctors benefiting financially from their relationship with pharmaceutical companies. Many doctors used to accept a reasonable consulting fee or speaker fee (and reasonable should remain defined as what is negotiated privately between the doctor and the company, not

The Physician Payments Sunshine Act

defined by the government or any third party) to give presentations at local restaurants with multiple local doctors to enjoy a reasonable meal and enjoy collegial interaction with colleagues while learning about updates on medical topics. The local economy would benefit from this steady flow of financial input into the community. The doctors attending would benefit because they would get valuable education with access to an expert and get to ask any kind of question to help them better serve their patients. The doctor presenting would benefit because of the valuable feedback regarding the information presented and because the financial reward would give him some buffer to then see additional free-care patients.

9. Because of section 6002 of the ACA, health care is more expensive, doctors learn less, doctors earn less, doctors spend more time working but less time on patient care, local restaurants have gone out of business or have fired workers, pharmaceutical representatives have lost their jobs or had to take pay cuts, all parties involved have had their lives needlessly complicated, erroneous defamatory information is permanently published with the inappropriate purpose to tarnish and shame doctors, and ultimately health care quality is not improved but is diminished. The additional irony is that I don't know any patient who is aware of this law, who utilizes the website or who even cares about this.

A sad side to this story is that certain doctors, particularly academic doctors, have been convinced (brainwashed) by their academic institutions that even talking to a pharmaceutical representative is an evil act. Many academic institutions and hospitals now forbid any of their doctors from being involved with pharmaceutical companies in any way. This serves no purpose but to harm medical research collaboration and educational collaboration. I have always found, with few exceptions, that pharmaceutical representatives provide extremely useful and timely information which helps doctors take care of patients.

10. The only solution is to completely eliminate this section of the law or eliminate the entire ACA.

Chapter Ten:

Health Care Fraud

1. There is a tremendous amount of money each year wasted on fraud and abuse in the health care system. One of the largest single factors impacting health care costs is fraud and abuse. If you consider just the federal government payments through the Medicare system, tens of billions of dollars per year are lost. Some of the ways the government has gone about addressing this subject are counterproductive.

2. Financial fraud and abuse in the health care system can result in civil and criminal actions – that is appropriate. However, not enough is being done to shut down the fraudsters. Not enough manpower is being devoted. Some of the anti-fraud strategies being enacted harm the legitimate medical doctors more than the fraudsters, and hence patient access to quality of care is diminished, not increased.

3. Unintended fraud and abuse: A medical doctor may be unable to keep up with the annual multifaceted changes of coding and billing and regulatory processes, and so the doctor inadvertently files claims with erroneous coding and gets paid differently than what he should. Ironically, this usually results in the doctor getting less than he is entitled to, but sometimes it results in his getting more. This is clearly unintentional and usually gets corrected in subsequent months.

4. Soft-core Fraud: This is more along the lines of abuse. A doctor might intentionally code for higher levels of service than was

warranted, or might do extra procedures that aren't absolutely necessary. This is hard to prove because the work is done, and it is a judgment call as to what is truly necessary. Some doctors actively engage in this behavior justified by the concept of occult compensation. Occult compensation, in this case, means that the doctor feels that the Medicare system or some other insurance system has been underpaying him and so he over utilizes the system to bring his total payments back in line with where he thinks they need to be for him to stay in business.

5. Hard-core fraud: There are so many types of hard-core fraud. This could be whereby a doctor bills and collects without even performing the services. This could be whereby someone who is not even a doctor pretends to be a doctor (either through identity theft or sham business) and bills and collects. This could be whereby someone is not a true medical doctor, but a paraprofessional clinician that tries to perform, and hence bill for, medical services that should be restricted to true allopathic medical doctors (imagine your barber gets to bill and collect for scalp botulinum toxin injections that he performed during your haircut session because of your headaches – after all he is "licensed"). Sometimes real companies find creative ways to fraudulently bill and collect.

6. One hypothetical example: Imagine a company that provides MRI imaging services for medical doctors to order for their patients. It seems straight forward, the doctor orders a brain MRI, the patient goes to the facility and gets put into the MRI machine, a technologist runs the equipment to obtain the images, then a radiologist M.D. reviews the images and writes a report for the referring medical doctor. The MRI company bills Medicare (or other insurance company) for the MRI services, and the

radiologist bills Medicare (or other insurance company) for the professional interpretation and report.

Fraud can occur in so many ways in this scenario. Imagine if the technologist does not turn on the equipment and the image used for the report is of someone else's brain (just the name was changed). Imagine that the MRI machine is just an elaborate cardboard box. Imagine that instead of an MRI machine, the technologist comes out with a camera and takes a picture of the person's head (the camera has a magnet in it and does produce an image). You can perhaps imagine several other iterations of fraud. This must be considered unlawful fraudulent activity, and any company that engages in this kind of behavior must not be paid – but it is possible, even likely, that they will be paid – over and over again to the tune of millions of dollars per year.

7. To further analyze this hypothetical example: For the sake of illustration, imagine the legitimate MRI company needs to collect a minimum of $1,000 per patient per order just to meet expenses and stay in business. Their billing results in collections of $1,200 per patient per order, so there is $200 profit. Imagine that the illegitimate MRI company needs only $200 per patient per order to meet expenses and stay in business, but they also collect $1,200. With that exorbitant extra profit, the illegitimate company's owners can quickly become wealthy and can afford to hire lawyers and consultants (and even lobbyists in some cases) that can help protect them and their profits and help perpetuate or even grow their scheme to multiple locations in multiple states.

8. It would seem logical to just shut down the illegitimate company or at least stop paying them. However, an example of how government officials might address this is when they say the following: "The cost of MRIs has gotten too high and so we are

going to cut the amount of money we pay to MRI facilities." The result is that, instead of paying $1,200 per MRI, they now pay only $600 per MRI. The government then publishes a report, while applauding themselves, stating that they have reduced the costs of MRIs to the taxpayer by 50%! The government agents smile and congratulate themselves over how they are now wasting less on fraud. It's true, they did save the taxpayers money, and they are spending less on fraud.

9. The problem is that now the legitimate MRI company goes out of business because the payment is lower than what it needs to stay in business – or at least they stop taking Medicare patients. The illegitimate company is still making $400 profit per MRI and so they stay in business. What's more, since there are fewer legitimate MRI companies available now, then more patients will be sent to the illegitimate companies. This has the ironic effect of increasing patient access to fraud and decreasing patient access to quality of care – all as a result of the government's ill-conceived method to decrease spending on fraud.

10. When medical doctors or professional medical organizations approach the government to help provide strategies to preserve appropriate fees but get rid of fraud, the government sometimes ignores such doctors and organizations. A reason the government often states as to why they will not shut down the illegitimate companies is their misuse of the concept of "restriction of trade." They fail to see health care services and fees as having a direct relationship to quality and authority of patient care – they see it merely as commerce. Therefore, one company providing the service is equal to any other company providing the service, and so they do not necessarily see the illegitimacy of the illegitimate company's practices and so the government concludes that it

doesn't want to "restrict trade." True restriction of trade would be if the government decided to pay one legitimate allopathic medical doctor and not pay another legitimate allopathic medical doctor for the exact same service. It is not restriction of trade to not pay a non-medical doctor when he tries to bill for allopathic medical services, and it is not restriction of trade to not pay when the billing is for sham services – but government officials (senators, congressman and officials at Medicare) seem unable to understand this and so refuse to effectively act on this.

Centers for Medicare and Medicaid Services [CMS] is controlled by Health and Human Services [HHS] which is controlled by the executive branch which is ultimately responsible for this. Senators and congressmen have means to intervene but they are usually unsuccessful. Commercial health insurance companies often just copy whatever happens in the Medicare system. I can write a thick book on this topic alone, but I think the point is made. The government and commercial insurers need to listen more to true allopathic medical doctors regarding fraud and abuse.

Chapter Eleven:

The Definition of a True American Medical Doctor

1. How are true American medical doctors defined, educated and trained? They start by achieving success in pursuit of a four year college degree. They score highly on medical school entrance exams. They are accepted through a competitive process to a medical school pursuant to a degree as a Medical Doctor, M.D., or a degree as a Doctor of Osteopathy, D.O. Medical school is typically four years with the first two years covering basic human health sciences including anatomy, physiology, neuroanatomy, neurophysiology, histology, pathology, organic chemistry, pharmacology, microbiology, immunology, nutrition, medical ethics, public health, and more.

There are national standardized exams after the first two years, and if the student does not pass, then the student is expelled and not allowed to continue. The final two years involve clinical rotations with hands-on experience in all of the clinical fields of medicine and surgery including internal medicine, general surgery, psychiatry, obstetrics, pediatrics, cardiology, neurology, and more. There is time allocated for electives such as additional focus on a particular clinical specialty or on research. There are national standardized exams again that must be passed otherwise the student is not allowed to graduate and not allowed to be awarded the M.D. or D.O. degree.

The Definition of a True American Medical Doctor

The current cost of college at this time may leave students with over $200,000.00 in debt with interest that continues to accrue while they are in medical school and further training. The cost of medical school is often more than that. The total debt for some medical school graduates at this time may exceed $500,000.00 with interest continuing to accrue nonstop, and the ability to make payments not coming until after fellowship training many years later. If the student fails out at any stage, the debt is still due.

2. The medical doctor then competes for a slot in internship and residency training programs. These can be highly competitive slots. Some specialties and some locations are more competitive than others. Sometimes slots are so uncompetitive that they go unfilled by American graduates and are offered to foreign medical graduates.

This fact is worthy of pause because, in some cases, foreign medical students do not have the appropriate level of training or appropriate cultural experience to be able to effectively practice medicine in the United States. There must be a greater effort to fill these slots with American graduates. Many of the foreign graduates have accumulated no debt due to free collegiate education and free medical school, so the Americans are often put at a relative financial disadvantage during residency training.

During the one year of internship, a medical doctor performs in the field of hospital-based internal medicine or in the field of hospital-based general surgery. Upon completion, the intern is required to take another national standardized exam. If the exam is passed, then the intern may be licensed as a medical doctor and can practice independently. It is rare for a doctor to stop at this level of training, but it most often occurs in the context of military doctors and in the context of doctors that want to become consultants or work in business or sales.

Most doctors continue on to residency training. This is more specialized. There are medical specialties such as cardiology, dermatology, pediatrics, infectious diseases, etc., and there are surgical specialties such as neurosurgery, orthopedic surgery, ophthalmology, etc. Residency programs are at least three years, but can be as long as seven years or more. It is common to do additional training in the form of fellowship training, which is at least one year but can be as much as three years. All told, after college, the typical medical doctor completes an additional eight to fourteen years of education and training, just to be able to practice independently. That's twelve to eighteen years beyond high school.

This long process weeds out the people who, for physical or psychological reasons, can't handle it. Society is left with naturally selected, strong, healthy, disease-resistant, dependable, reliable, talented, functional, almost machines of individuals to serve faithfully for the rest of their lives as true American medical doctors.

Today, applicants for medical schools are not necessarily chosen for their likelihood to succeed, but are chosen based on filling quotas for skin color, gender, ethnicity, religion, political affiliation, likeliness to cooperate with those in authority or due to friendships, attractiveness or other inappropriate subjective reasons. Many of the weak ones, when they are failing or falling apart, are propped up with exemptions or special programs. Our society is experiencing the dumbing down and feebling of the American doctor. The doctors of today are far less competent, intelligent, reliable, functional, disease-resistant or talented compared to doctors of past decades.

Phraseology regarding health care personnel can get confusing. Here are some clarifications: A health care clinician is any person working with patients. A health care provider is any person working with patients. A health care practitioner is any person working with patients. An academic doctor is a person primarily engaged in teaching. A scientist or a researcher doctor is a person primarily engaged in research. A clinical doctor is person primarily engaged in patient care. The word "medicine" is a noun and refers to medication. The phrase "the practice of medicine" refers to the act of providing allopathic medical doctor intervention for diagnosis and treatment of illness, injury or degeneration. The word "physician" refers to an allopathic medical doctor who focuses on using medicinal treatments (and not surgical treatments) – but that word has been losing its meaning. The word "surgeon" refers to an allopathic medical doctor who focuses on using surgical intervention. Below are further health care personnel clarifications.

It is important to be clear about the difference between physicians and surgeons. True physicians are allopathic medical doctors who focus on using medicinal and therapeutic means to treat illness, injury or degeneration. Surgeons are true allopathic medical doctors who focus on using surgical techniques to treat illness, injury or degeneration. Physicians can practice in a broad range of settings, mostly outpatient (non-hospital), but surgeons must practice within the context of a hospital or surgical facility setting. One additional difference is that surgeons spend most of their patient encounter with the patient unconscious – and so their perspective needs to be understood in that context. The word "physician" has been stolen by alternative care practitioners and has lost its intended meaning. For perfect clarity, we must say "allopathic medical doctor physicians," or words to that effect.

2. The best clinical medical doctors, in training, choose the most difficult clinical rotations and immerse themselves into clinical work non-stop during medical school, internship, residency and fellowship. This is their once in a lifetime opportunity to get exposure to the full breadth and depth of clinical medicine and surgery. This also represents a closing window of opportunity to build a solid foundation of clinical excellence which will define the quality of their future as medical doctors. The worst clinical doctors minimize their clinical involvement at this stage and pursue research rotations instead. To be clear, the phrase "clinical medical doctor" refers to a medical doctor who focuses on patient care instead of teaching (as with academic medical doctors) or research (as with medical doctor scientists).

3. There has been the unfortunate rise of the "M.D.-Ph.D. Program." This is when a medical doctor combines the pursuit of the medical degree along with the pursuit of a degree in basic science research. In my professional opinion, this has distracted the medical community away from its primary purpose, has caused the leaders of the medical profession to abdicate their authority and influence over clinical health care, and has shifted the culture of medical doctoring away from patient care for the sake of research. To be clear, I am not diminishing the importance of health research. I am pointing out that medical doctors are now focusing on research at the expense of patient care. Ph.D. researchers who want to do human medical research must be supported and encouraged, but for that researcher to also get the

M.D. degree, and take a valuable training slot away from someone who would have gone on to be a clinic medical doctor, is counterproductive toward solving the medical doctor shortage crisis we are facing in America today.

Instead, medical schools and subsequent training programs will be much improved if they include courses on the business of medicine, on helping doctors to set up and run private practices, on helping doctors keep up with and comply with billing, coding, administrative and regulatory issues, on helping doctors to understand and comply with legal issues and engage in legislative lobbying, on helping doctors manage finance issues such as paying down their school loan debt and how to negotiate financial contracts with insurance companies and others. This shift of emphasis will enable greater opportunities for health care innovation.

4. Internship and residency training programs are unnecessarily paid for by the federal government through Medicare even though private hospitals, non-profit hospitals and academic institutions "profit" from the labor of those doctors-in-training. It is estimated that the federal government is unnecessarily spending more than ten billion dollars annually on this. Furthermore, most residency training programs are inefficient regarding clinical training. Any three year residency program could be completed more efficiently in two years, any five year program in three, and any seven year program in four. What's more, the residency programs could be converted into apprenticeship programs which could take place within the context of community-based private practices. Most medical care, especially non-surgical, takes place in the outpatient community setting, but internship and residency training, as

currently configured, takes place within hospital settings. Ironically, with the way current residency programs are set up, the most useful and comprehensive learning takes place in the first year or two AFTER the doctor leaves the program. It takes place while the doctor is employed as a junior attending under the tutelage of more senior doctors in the practice that he joins. If the doctor graduates a residency program and has the bad fortune of staying on at an academic medical center, without some years spent in a private practice, then that doctor will never have the opportunity to be fully trained or fully competent in his field. Unfortunately, this is the current trend.

5. Continuing medical education [CME] is essential for all medical doctors to keep up with evolving knowledge and technology. This is appropriate because if left to rely on information obtained in medical school and residency, most doctors would suffer from obsolete knowledge in as little as five to ten years. I suggest that medical doctors pursue CME in a broad range of topics each year and not limit themselves to a single specialty area as is often the case.

6. The requirement of board certification is a myth. With the rise of specialties and subspecialties, and the rise of fellowship training programs, so has risen the concept of board certification. Somehow, even though medical doctors have successfully completed their comprehensive training, and have successfully completed their exams, and have fulfilled their licensing and credentialing requirements, a group of doctors, arrogant old men, formed organizations (like exclusive clubs) and appointed themselves as the deciders and dictators over all knowledge in their chosen field, for example, neurology. They then created the concept of having doctors, for example, neurologists, pay them

exorbitant sums of money for the privilege of taking unreasonable tests (from which the arrogant old men who formed the board gave themselves and their friends lifetime exemptions). Only if that doctor paid that organization that fee and passed that unreasonable test, then could he say that he was "board-certified." The boards were established by collusion whereby there could be only one board for each specialty and the pursuant subspecialties – to eliminate competition for the sake of financial monopoly. The concept of board certification must be done away with. Unfortunately, some institutions such as hospitals and insurance companies still ask to see such certificates.

As if board certification wasn't enough of a monopolistic scam perpetrated on medical doctors, the next generation of people who took over the boards came up with the concept of maintenance of certification [MOC]. This then put a time limit on the board certification such that after so many years the doctors had to pay the exorbitant fees again, and take unreasonable tests again, and jump through several other weird nonsensical hoops to be able to continue to say they are board certified. At this time it is appropriate for all doctors to ignore MOC – it has absolutely no meaning. At this time it is appropriate for all institutions, including hospitals and insurance companies to ignore the concept of MOC. If the boards do not cease the MOC concept, then doctors should definitely create alternative organizations which will charge lower fees, adopt more appropriate assessment methods and award lifetime certifications.

7. Professional medical organizations are the best source for doctors and surgeons to seek continuing education and practice guidance. These organizations provide a broad spectrum of educational options from clinical to academic to scientific. The

organizations recruit a good mix of academic and private practice educators across a broad geographic and even international perspective. Many of these organizations have been hijacked by academia and so their utility has diminished and their educational presentations have become increasingly biased and censored (against clinical practice and against private practice, while being pro academic and pro scientific research) – but these venues are still the best options for educational opportunities.

Some state medical societies and their subsidiaries can be very helpful to medical doctors for continuing education and practice guidance. Membership numbers in such organizations have greatly diminished over recent years, and hence their funding has likewise diminished.

8. The meaning of the title of doctor has been eroded over time due to "credential creep," "degree inflation" and the medical-doctor-wannabe syndrome. Today, the only doctors that are true allopathic medical doctors are those with an M.D. degree (Medical Doctor), with appropriate subsequent training and licensure, or those with a D.O. degree (Doctor of Osteopathy), with appropriate subsequent training and licensure. All other care practitioners are not true allopathic medical doctors, but are people who "identify" as medical doctors – sometimes known as medical-doctor-wannabes. In general, these medical-doctor-wannabes are innocuous. In some cases they can cause medical harm. In some cases they are a significant source of health care insurance fraud and abuse – adding substantial unnecessary cost to the health care system.

These alternative care practitioners achieve the title of "doctor" by getting a "doctorate" degree, Ph.D., or by creating or maintaining some organization that confers some form of alternative "doctor" degree and license, but not an M.D. or D.O. With the title of "doctor" or some other currently acceptable "health care practitioner" title, they obtain their authority, not through the legitimate ranks of the traditional allopathic medical community, but through lobbying, legislating and litigating. It would seem obvious that a patient would want a "doctor" to diagnose and treat him because the doctor was appropriately educated and trained and licensed, not because the "doctor" and his organization lobbied and paid politicians to create legislative decrees or because the "doctor" sued or litigated for judge's rulings to force society to allow this non-medical-doctor "doctor" or "health care practitioner" to be inserted into the health care system with some false sense of equivalency to true allopathic medical doctors.

The medical-doctor-wannabes have creatively tried to model their organizations (but not their training) on the organizations of true allopathic medical doctors. And so they have licensing bodies and board certification bodies and now they have increased their level of mimicking by litigating and legislating or otherwise just stealing the right to call themselves "physicians." Prior to recent years this was one of the last titles true medical doctors could use to distinguish themselves from non-medical doctors, so these practitioners went after that and so the word "physician" is now confusing. Such practitioners are going even further. They know that true medical doctors have specialty categories such as neurologist, cardiologist, gastroenterologist, sports physician, etc. Such practitioners are now litigating and legislating or otherwise just stealing the right to call themselves these names as well.

To be fair, many such practitioners are wonderful caring individuals that genuinely desire to help people, and genuinely do help people. Most focus on the art of caring, with a reasonable understanding of human nature. This does not change the fact that there are some among them who inappropriately try to practice allopathic health care or perform tests and procedures well beyond the scope of their education, knowledge, training and authority. This adds tremendous cost to the American health care system, because in most cases, the patient with a true medical diagnosis will ultimately need to see a true medical doctor and that true medical doctor will have to repeat all the tests in a more valid and reliable way. As a result the health care costs double or triple.

The most common cases of medical-doctor-wannabe syndrome may be found among some chiropractors, naturopathic practitioners and homeopathic practitioners. They title themselves D.C. or N.D. or H.D. or N.MD. or D.Ht. or DHANP or CCH, etc. Their schools and training, beyond high school, can be as little as four to five years total (compared to total of twelve to eighteen years for true allopathic medical doctors). Entry into such schools does not even require obtaining a college degree as a prerequisite in some cases. Much of their training focuses on marketing, business administration, legislative lobbying and litigating in some cases.

Such practitioners are regulated on a state level. There are some states that appropriately understand the strict limitations that must be placed on such practitioners, and limit them accordingly – or exclude them entirely. There are some states that do not understand this, either due to ignorance of their legislators and regulators or possibly because such practitioners have spent enough money lobbying and litigating to win over the judges and legislators. In those unfortunate states, such practitioners may be given inappropriate authority. If you live in such a state, I suggest you move to a more advanced state, your life might depend on it.

9. Nurse Practitioners [N.P.s] and Physicians Assistants [P.A.s] are considered "physician extenders" working under the authority of true medical doctors. N.P.s and P.A.s are now inexorably interwoven into the fabric of the American health care system, and they do provide substantial benefit. They have become most valuable in situations where they have achieved substantial on-the-job training and experience well beyond their basic degree program – and where they remain under the leadership of a true medical doctor. Due to premeditated credential creep and degree inflation techniques at some N.P. and P.A. training programs, these practitioners are now awarded the "doctorate" degree for the specific purpose of intending such practitioners to be called "doctor."

Due to premeditated credential creep and degree inflation techniques now some physical therapy training programs award the "doctorate" degree for the specific purpose of intending such therapist to be called "doctor." Next you will have to call your massage therapist "doctor." Eventually you will have to call the nurse's aide who changes your bedpan in the hospital "doctor" (of bedpanology). I suspect the doctor-wannabe-syndrome will spread so far and wide that there will be a one week online course, at the cost of $100, to award the title of "doctor" without even the basic requirement of a high school diploma.

I know the following statement is offensive, but it is a truth that must be revealed: Even with their multiple levels of comprehensive screening, even with their many years of selfless dedication, servitude, education and training, and even with their multiple layers of credentialing processing, many of the true allopathic medical doctors, M.D.s and D.O.s, as physicians and surgeons today, are either borderline incompetent or completely incompetent. So what entitles anyone to believe that we can take people who are far less well-educated and far less well-trained, and expect them to be sufficient "doctors?"

It is crucial to understand that hospitals, medical centers, pharmaceutical companies, pharmacies, Medicare, health insurance companies and health care organizations do not provide health care. Allopathic medical doctors provide health care. All other health care personnel provide health care under the ultimate guidance of allopathic medical doctors. You can remove almost any person or place or thing from the health care system, but if you still have the true allopathic medical doctor and the patient, then you have a health care system. If you remove the allopathic medical doctor or the patient, even if you have every other person and place and thing, then you do not have a health care system.

10. Historically, true medical doctors would complete all of their training and then either join a private practice group or initiate an independent private practice. They would have a medical office in the community and would have "privileges" at a nearby hospital to be able to take care of their patients when hospitalized. Medical doctors of the past were more intelligent, more self-sufficient, had strong character, had leadership ability, and were dedicated to serving patients and the community.

The Definition of a True American Medical Doctor

Today, many doctors, upon finishing their training, avoid private practice or avoid the clinical practice of medicine as much as possible. Many prefer to be employed by a hospital or health care organization. Many prefer that hospital or that health care organization to have an academic medical school or university affiliation. Many prefer to do research and not be involved in patient care. Many tend to have an over-inflated self-assessment of their own abilities since the current culture of the medical profession tells them that academic doctors who spend most time on teaching or research are the smart talented ones, and the community doctors who spend most time on clinical patient care are the dumb useless ones. Ironically, it is the academic, teaching and researching medical doctors that are most likely to be clinically impotent, yet they will be promoted by their organizations as the thought leaders of our day.

Many academic researching medical doctors have a strong need to be defined by something bigger than themselves. They cannot conceive of practicing alone in the community and saying to their patient, "I am Dr. Johnson, and I dedicate my life to taking care of you and others like you." However, they will take great pride in saying to their patient (on the rare occasions that they see a patient) something to the following effect: "As you know, I am a Greatstone General Hospital University Professor, therefore you know that you are getting access to one of the greatest doctors in the world." Yes, this sort of thing really does happen often. Many do not see themselves as having become a doctor to be able to serve and help patients. Instead many are motivated by the desire to please their academic employer, to pursue titles such as director or chief or chairman and define themselves by the prestige associated with the place they work. Many spend their lives devoted to building monuments to themselves such as creating a university endowed chair in their own name. Many are motivated to become an assistant professor then associate professor then full professor. Many are motivated to get their name published in as many medical journals as possible, regardless of the usefulness or validity of the research. Many care about the appearance of things, not the substance of things. Many want to be admired, revered and famous. Even though they have so much to learn, they just want to teach, and, as they teach, they propagate their ignorance and inflated attitude to the next generation of medical doctors. Just as ironic, they will pursue this path even if they get paid one half or one quarter of what they could earn in private practice. Many doctors have become procedure performers, consult performers, opinion renderers and prescription givers instead of problem solvers, healers and care providers.

Medical doctors have become notoriously poor businessmen and poor participants in legal, legislative and political processes. This abdication of community leadership, authority and responsibility has been exploited by third parties. This, in turn, has given rise to the American health care system being overrun by special interests such as insurance companies, pharmaceutical companies, biomedical technology companies, hospitals, medical centers, health care organizations, big business, lawyers, politicians, and non-medical-doctor care-providers. Medical doctors are more interested in fighting with other medical doctors over who will be the next chief or director or chairman of this hospital program or that committee, etc., than they are about the big picture outside of their little world. They don't recognize that we are in the process of total destruction of

The Definition of a True American Medical Doctor

the American health care system – a system that they should have been presiding over and protecting.

Many medical doctors of today are like ants wrestling each other over a crumb while being carried on the tongue of an anteater to their own demise. They just don't get it.

Chapter Twelve:

Ranking and Rating Medical Doctors

1.   There is no company or website I know of that can appropriately or correctly rank or rate or otherwise assess the competency of any medical doctor.

2.   There are many doctor-rating website businesses and many are well funded.   Many have achieved preferential status on search engines, most likely through financial compensation to the search provider.   It is amazing that when you do an internet search for a particular medical doctor, at least ten doctor-rating sites will come up first.   It may be quite a struggle to find that doctor's website or office location or hospital affiliation or board of medicine profile – all of the things you were probably looking for when you entered the doctor's name in the search.

3.   People who are disgruntled are most likely to visit a rating website and enter a review; clearly in an attempt to defame the doctor.   A medical doctor could do perfectly well with over 30,000 patients, and poorly with two.   Those two will write seventeen negative reviews.   Of the 30,000, maybe three will write positive reviews.

4.   I know of rating websites that will, as a default, give a doctor a poor rating and then contact that doctor stating something to this effect: "We see that you have a poor rating on our website, if you will just become a member, login and provide certain information, we can assure you that your rating will improve..." It is a scam to get the doctor to participate and add legitimacy to

that company and hence convince investors that the company has many members and is worthy of investment capital. Most doctor's egos are easily bruised and so they are often taken advantage of in such situations.

5. People who write negative reviews against doctors are often not patients but "competitors." One doctor who wants to diminish the reputation of another nearby doctor, in competition for fame and patients, will spend the time, pretending to be a patient, posting negative reviews about his competitor.

6. People who write negative reviews against doctors are often not patients but (former) employees or (former) friends or family members who are upset for some reason and see this as an easy way to take a shot.

7. People who write negative reviews against doctors are sometimes patients who were unable to get what they wanted from the doctor. For example, some patients like to have opioid prescriptions so they can sell the pills on the street for profit. If the doctor says no, then the patient can threaten the following: "I'll post multiple negative reviews about you on every website I can get my hands on if you don't do what I want..." You can imagine other similar examples.

8. People who write positive reviews about doctors are often not patients but the doctor himself and his staff. Some doctors monitor such websites and participate aggressively to skew the appearance as very positive, regardless of truth. Also, be suspicious of major magazine publications of "Best Doctors" or words to that effect. Many such rankings are usually publicity stunts or involve payments or involve a voting system whereby the doctor can vote for himself a thousand times and ask all his

friends to vote for him a thousand times (in reciprocity for his voting for them), or involve some other manipulative strategy that has little to do with "best." This concept often applies to "Best Hospitals" listings as well.

9. The best way to get information about a doctor is to go to his website, go to his profile on an affiliated hospital website, go to the board of medicine website of the state in which the doctor practices, talk to his staff, talk to referring physicians and by word of mouth from other patients (knowing that the vast majority of patients do not post reviews on websites).

10. If you have a problem with a doctor or a doctor's office, the first venue to seek correction is through that doctor's office. Speak with the practice manager to explain the problem. Write a letter directed confidentially to the doctor. Provide meaningful feedback to help the doctor improve his practice, improve his office conditions and improve his staff interactions. Doctors will value this kind of feedback and be very willing to improve, unless the request is too unreasonable (or unethical or unlawful).

Chapter Thirteen:

Onsite and Remote Health Care

1. It would make for a more healthful society if health care could be accessed onsite at various public buildings or at various remote locations, at least of an emergent or urgent care nature. This may be the case already in some instances, but inconsistently at best. This concept must be made into a new standard of access to care.

2. All public airports must include an onsite medical facility and include a quarantine section. Air travel is always stressful and more so recently. Issues such as myocardial infarction (heart attack), cerebral infarct (stroke), deep vein thrombosis, pulmonary embolism, acute headaches, acute gastrointestinal issues, shortness of breath, fainting, seizures, anxiety, panic, injury from violence and even serious infections are all issues that may be more rapidly and efficiently addressed onsite, either pre-security checkpoint or post-security checkpoint. Access to the facility would be for travelers as well as airport workers. Lives can be saved if this is implemented. It could be contracted with a private practice group so specialized, it can be contracted with a nearby hospital or the airport can hire medical doctors directly to run the facility. Payment for the services would be commensurate with systems currently in place at other emergency care and urgent care facilities, or could be paid for implementation of an airport health transit fee, or something to that effect, as new form of travel insurance. Regarding international travelers, there must be a requirement for purchasing short term health care insurance.

3. Prison health care is problematic. There are some prison health care facilities in the United States that are wonderful and successful. However, for the most part, prison health care is inadequate or even harmful. Some might argue that people in prison have made choices in their life that cause them to forfeit the privilege of access to quality health care or even forfeit access to any health care. However, the winning ethical argument is that prisoners, especially in cases of unknown guilt or innocence, must be treated as any other human being patient in America, with kindness, dignity, respect and timely access to appropriate medical care. Criminal activity is often a medical or psychiatric diagnosis. In many cases medical conditions may inadvertently result in what appears to be criminal activity: an acute psychotic break, a reaction to recreational drugs, a seizure, a sleep disorder, a reaction to a prescribed medication, etc. Most criminals need treatment not punishment.

Each prison must have an appropriate health care medical facility, staffed by appropriately qualified medical doctors, addiction experts, dentists, nutritionists and psychiatric staff, available to all inmates. The facility must be inspected and regulated, like any other hospital or medical facility, to maintain cleanliness, safety and current technology.

The prison itself must be run as a medical rehabilitation facility. American prisons of today are better classified as school grounds for training inmates in how to be more successful criminals. American prisons of today are places where inmate on inmate violence is too common and authority figures are sometimes involved in inmate abuse of every type imaginable. Not only does society need to be protected from dangerous criminals, but inmates need to be protected from each other, protected from the negative influences they might have on each other, and protected so they can have a chance to heal (otherwise known as reform). Yes, I understand, some criminals will never heal (reform), but that does not mean we should give up on the rest, if at least to minimize recidivism. We need to understand not just the criminal mind but the criminal brain. We need to explore and develop medical and surgical techniques to cure various types of criminality. We need to develop technology to be able to diagnose medical or genetic predispositions toward types of criminality – before there are victims, police, judges and jails involved.

4. Athletic arenas usually have ambulance transport available for emergencies. Sometimes people fall and get injured, sometimes people have a heart attack or stroke, often the athletes get injured. Some arenas have an onsite medical treatment room with some sutures and bandages. To be considered a state of the art athletic arena, the arena must have a robust emergency care facility. It may be staffed only during events or, better, it could be a full time facility having a dual role also serving the local community. There needs to be two types of access. One for the spectators, employees, general public, etc., and one separate for the athletes. Triage and observational capabilities will be crucial. Efficient linking to nearby tertiary care hospital will be essential (physically via unobstructed ambulance transport and electronically via telemedicine). There will need to be staff in place, and infrastructure in place, to help the potential patients to be moved through the arena to the care facility.

5. Shopping malls and convention centers and the like could do well to have at least one urgent care facility which has efficient linking to nearby tertiary care hospital (physically via

unobstructed ambulance transport and electronically via telemedicine). There may need to be staff in place to help the potential patients to be moved through the mall or center to the care facility.

6. In deserts throughout the country (and ultimately throughout the world) the government(s) could provide a valuable service by maintaining a health grid such that, for example, every ten square miles there will be a location to house a water supply, basic first aid materials, communication capabilities, appropriate shelter for temporary use by lost or injured or ill travelers – and some sort of beacon to mark its location. This would be problematic on private land, but would be reasonable on public land.

7. In forests or mountains throughout the country (and ultimately throughout the world) the government(s) could provide a valuable service by maintaining a health grid such that, for example, every ten square miles there will be a location to house a water supply, basic first aid materials, communication capabilities, appropriate shelter for temporary use by lost or injured or ill travelers – and some sort of beacon to mark its location. This would be problematic on private land, but would be reasonable on public land.

8. In frozen or tundra lands throughout the country (and ultimately throughout the world) the government(s) could provide a valuable service by maintaining a health grid such that, for example, every ten square miles for the first 200 miles off shore and then more sparsely thereafter, there will be a location to house a water supply, basic first aid materials, communication capabilities, appropriate shelter for temporary use by lost or injured or ill travelers – and some sort of beacon to mark its

location. This would be problematic on private land, but would be reasonable on public land.

9. In large water bodies throughout the country off coast (and ultimately throughout the world) the government(s) could provide a valuable service by maintaining a health grid such that, for example, every ten square miles there will be a location to house a water supply, basic first aid materials, communication capabilities, appropriate shelter for temporary use by lost or injured or ill travelers – and some sort of beacon to mark its location. This would be challenging in oceans, but not impossible.

10. At intervals along each international border and certainly at border control stations, the government could provide a valuable service by maintaining health screening and quarantining facilities. The primary purpose would be to protect the citizens of the United States from potentially contagious illnesses and parasites and potentially toxic substances. The secondary purpose would be to provide a safe house for those who are crossing the border underage or otherwise at risk of harm or death in the wilderness.

Chapter Fourteen:

Institutions and Industries of Health Care

1. The pharmaceutical industry and biomedical technology companies play crucial roles in modern health care. Without the billions of dollars of research conducted each year and without the thousands of products currently available, millions of patients each year would be suffering more and dying younger. However, the cost analysis associated with research, development, clinical trials, legal liability, FDA approval, marketing, distribution, and patent limitations is becoming increasingly unsustainable. There may be a miracle drug available for a certain condition, but if the price per pill is too high, then it is as if it didn't exist.

One potential solution is to change the drug patent concept to one resembling a hybrid between trademark and trade secret. Products that are protected by trademark or trade secret cannot be copied and the infringement protection is indefinite. With a drug patent, it is conceivable that the time it takes to bring the drug to market will be longer than the patent will be protected from infringement on the market. The pharmaceutical company may spend billions of dollars on drugs that ultimately don't make it to market, and so the costs of these failures must be added to the costs of the drugs that do make it. Since there is a relatively short window, the prices must be high to compensate and allow for future research. If every success is allowed to remain like a hybrid of trademark and trade secret, then there will be no such thing as generics and the prices of the brand name drugs will not have to be so high because the companies can profit for decades, not just years, from each drug.

Another potential solution is to speed up the FDA approval time frame. An additional potential solution is to force the FDA to bear the brunt of liability. How is it that the FDA will approve a drug for efficacy and safety but when lawyers find some way to convince a judge that a drug is unsafe, the company itself bears the liability? The FDA must be equally liable or entirely liable since the FDA is the authority that approves the products for market. A better potential solution is to have a no-fault insurance program to compensate patients related to pharmaceutical or biomedical technology mishaps. The payments will not need to involve lawyers or lawsuits.

Biomedical technology companies are ones that develop diagnostic and treatment products including imaging technology, surgically implanted artificial joints, genetic testing, genetic engineering, pure biological products such as vaccines, blood products, bodily tissues, and so on. These biotechnological products are considered more responsible than anything else for the increased costs in the American health care system.

Some of these pharmaceutical and biomedical technology companies are influential with their billions of dollars leveraged by their teams of lawyers and lobbyists. They tend to be good at manipulating all ends of the health care system to assure profits. More than any other factor, health care insurance money is being diverted away from medical doctors' salaries to give the money to these companies. The average employee at a pharmaceutical or biomedical technology company makes more money than the average employee in the clinical health care field (which includes medical doctors).

2.   Hospitals are absolutely necessary institutions in any community; however, they have gained too much influence and control over the business of health care. In the mind of many hospital administrators, the hospital does not exist for the benefit of the community, doctors and patients. Instead they believe the community, doctors and patients exist for the benefit of the hospital. Doctors have traditionally maintained an adversarial relationship with hospitals as doctors have honorably understood the potential for a horrible conflict of interest. However, many doctors, for the sake of convenience or laziness, have dishonorably given in to being employed by hospitals. This has given non-doctors control over doctors and patients and health care: namely hospital administrators and big business entities. Hospitals have grown too big, have merged and bought up smaller hospitals and medical practices to form "health care organizations." This has led to the emergence of mini monopolies which exist for the primary benefit of the health care organization business entity to gain influence over money and gain control over information and people.

These mini monopolies need to be busted up, and certificate of need regulations must be abolished in states that still have such regulations. New entities must have no barriers to compete with the well-established facilities: this will accelerate innovation, increase choices and drive prices down.

Patients would be better served with smaller independent hospitals and surgical centers and urgent care centers spaced according to population density throughout a region. Few medical doctors should be direct employees of hospitals. Hospitals and other health care facilities must be restricted to ownership by allopathic medical doctors. Most of the money that comes into a hospital comes from the work of the allopathic medical doctors (except for the parking garage, the gift shop and the cafeteria). Without doctors there would be no hospitals. However, hospitals, medical centers and health care organizations spend lavishly on fancy corporate buildings, pay non-doctor administrators obscenely high salaries, sometimes hire more administrators than doctors, pay their medical doctor employees below going rates, and waste money on websites, newsletters, committees and meetings. The wasted money for all that corporate fun comes from patient care. I could write a book on this topic alone, but at least you get a hint.

Large health care organizations, large medical centers and hospital conglomerates need to be disbanded due to antitrust concerns, but this is not happening. The opposite is the trend at this time. There is less competition and there are fewer independent medical doctors. This seriously harms patients, the medical profession and the American health care system.

Health care is not a product like hamburgers, but that's how it's being treated. You can have a restaurant facility crank out hamburgers, made of a certain formula, performed by anybody with minimal training, and you will easily achieve a consistent outcome. However, you can have a health care facility crank out medical doctor patient care visits, even following specific algorithms, guidelines and protocols by highly trained medical doctors, and you will never achieve a consistent outcome. Unfortunately, doctors are not interchangeable (some are good clinicians and some are not). Patients, even those carrying the same diagnosis, are all unique and each requires a custom approach. Therefore, the current model implemented by the large health care conglomerates whereby administrators dictate committee-designed algorithms, guidelines and protocols to their medical doctors (which they assume to be interchangeable – after all how hard could it be to just follow the algorithms?), and expect that all patients will be appropriately served, is intolerably flawed and failing.

3.   Commercial health insurance companies have become important third parties in the health care financial equation. However, they are dictated to by federal and state governments, and they in turn dictate to local medical doctors and hospitals.

They may be able to dictate payment policies to the doctor because the doctor has the free will to contract with that company or not. However, they must never be allowed to dictate patient care decisions to the doctor, as they now often do – this is the equivalent of a company practicing medicine without a license. They must adapt their business to the needs of the doctor and the needs of the patient and not the other way around as it is currently configured. If you could only see the amount of people that work in the insurance industry, how much money is spent on these employees, and on the magnificent real estate they own or lease, then consider how much profit these companies make – it would make you wonder how much money is being wasted on these third party middlemen.

We must return to the complete free market economy of health care, without the middlemen. Medical doctor private practices and hospitals must be forced to live with only what the market will bear. Pharmaceutical and biomedical technology companies will charge less per product because the patients will pay directly – no more faceless third party payers with huge budgets. There will be no waste and little fraud. Patients will have decreased access to health care in general, but will reserve that access for only when necessary and the access will be more to high quality and less to fraud or incompetence. The concept of prevention will become more valuable as people will be forced to live more healthy lifestyles and take on more personal responsibility. Society in general will be strengthened and toughened. The American health care system will be much simpler and more successful.

4. Industries now try to get involved in patient care management. It is common for pharmaceutical companies, pharmacies and health insurance companies to reach out to patients either on the phone or in writing attempting to guide their health care related to certain diagnoses – this is absurd and dangerous. For example, a company representative might call a patient and say something to the following effect: "We see that you carry the diagnosis of multiple sclerosis, we would like to make sure your doctor has made you aware of this or that..." and the information may be completely wrong, or at least inappropriate for that patient, and amounts to companies or individuals at those companies practicing medicine without a license and interfering with patient care.

5. Some Vitamin and nutraceutical manufacturers make obscene profits with products of dubious value or with potentially harmful contents. Many over the counter nutritional supplements make marketing claims to treat or cure medical problems but then, in the fine print, state that their products cannot be used to treat or cure any medical problem. These products are minimally regulated, and so they, at times, do not even have to contain in the pills exactly what is written on the label. This is problematic

for several reasons. The substance may be inert and not provide the stated supplement in an absorbable form, and so a deficient patient goes on being deficient. The substance may be toxic to some degree, and hence potentially harmful to the patient. The substance may be combined with other substances in one pill, and so when combined with the patient's prescription medications, a malabsorption or other harmful effect could occur. Additionally, the cost of the substance might be pennies, but the price to the patient may be twenty or a hundred dollars.

6. The internet search engines and health care related websites, even those websites of governmental agencies or academic institutions, have unreliable, false or conflicting information. It is NOT POSSIBLE at this point in history to get consistently valid, reliable, accurate, timely, truthful, appropriate medical or health care information on the internet. The trend toward false, biased, conflicting, commercial-motivated information is increasing, and the percentage of valid, reliable and accurate information is decreasing. Patients who search health care information on the internet will be steered toward either inappropriate commercial products or misleading information which will increase their fear, or else wind up on a webpage that exists purely for the purpose of bringing in advertising dollars for the website owner. Patients will do best to consult with an appropriately trained true clinical allopathic medical doctor to have all their questions answered. If that doctor does not take the time to satisfactorily answer the questions, find one that will and stick with him.

7. Medical apps, applications or programs for computers and other electronic devices, smart phones and gadgets, are popular. These are mostly conversational pieces for their users, and profit centers for their makers. It is extremely doubtful, at this time,

that there are any apps that validly, reliably and accurately serve the purpose for which they are intended. At this point in history, if you are using a medical app, use it for fun like it's a game unless specifically directed and coordinated by a true allopathic medical doctor.

8.   Medical colleges may be stand-alone institutions or a subsidiary of some university system. These medical colleges will be affiliated with one or more hospitals. The medical doctors that are employed by, or affiliated with, such a medical college or university hospital system will have what is known as an academic appointment. There is an academic hierarchical structure. The medical students are at the lowest level, then interns, then residents and then fellows – these are levels of training. Upon completion of training, the hierarchy continues to junior attending doctors, senior attending doctors, program directors, division chiefs, department chairs, chief medical officers or some equivalent title and then Deans. Superimposed on this structure is an additional hierarchy of educational titles starting with instructor, then assistant professor, then associate professor and then full professor. To think that the medical world in the practice of medicine tries to imitate the academic world with its hierarchies is laughable, counterproductive, anti-innovative and must be abolished. It serves no purpose other than to distract medical doctors away from patient care responsibilities and diminishes their patient-care excellence.

Too often, in the setting of academic facilities, patients have become the play things of ineffective medical intellectual doctors – I call them ineffectuals or IMIDs.

9. Professional medical associations and state medical societies are relatively unbiased valuable resources for medical doctors.

Such organizations typically still hold the doctors' and the patients' best interests as priority. They provide ongoing collegial education programs, practice support programs and advocacy programs. Some of these also have a lobbying component. I encourage medical doctors to join, utilize and be supportive of such organizations and also to be generously supportive of their lobbying components. These organizations remain the best hope for unbiased continuing medical education, for doctor and patient advocacy and for emerging power to effect positive legislative change.

10. The government: I could write an encyclopedia just to outline the government's involvement in health care – considering the federal, state, county and city levels. Some of it is extremely important and helpful to American citizens: the Center for Disease Control and Prevention [CDC], the National Institutes of Health [NIH], the Food and Drug Administration [FDA], the Office of the Inspector General [OIG], the departments of public health, the departments of children and families, the boards of medicine, etc. Some of it is useless or even harmful to American citizens.

Aside from military health care which is provided to active duty under the Department of Defense and to veterans under the Veterans Administration, most federal health care regulatory authority falls under the jurisdiction of the Department of Health and Human Services [HHS] and its multiple divisions and agencies. HHS is led by a cabinet-level secretary which is usually a political operative of the President, but should be an unbiased clinical allopathic medical doctor. There have been a couple of cases of medical doctors serving in this role, but I believe the M.D. degree with prior clinical experience must be a minimum requirement.

Institutions and Industries of Health Care

On the federal level, HHS incorporates the following divisions and agencies: ACF, ACL, AHRQ, ATSDR, ASA, ASFR, ASGA, ASH, ASL, ASPE, ASPR, ASPA, CDC, CMS, DAB, FDA, HRSA, IOS, IHS, NIH, OCR, OIG, OIEA, OMHA, OGC, ONC, and SAMHSA. Each state has its own spectrum of health care regulatory divisions and agencies. The same goes for major counties and cities. This is all in addition to federal mandates, executive actions and acts and laws of Congress. This is all in addition to state mandates, executive actions and acts and laws of state legislatures; and so on for county and city levels.

It is worth providing a brief overview of the Centers for Medicare and Medicaid Services [CMS] division of HHS. The most important message is that this is the single most influential force driving the direction of the American health care system today, and it is run by people who are not elected by the citizenry and who are rarely held accountable for their actions in any way by anyone. Furthermore, they can do almost anything they want with the system at any time and their actions effectively rule by decree, with no viable options to modify them other than by a successful act of Congress (which rarely happens). By the nature of its essentially unchecked authority and control over the American health care system, this organization needs to be disbanded. Medicare and Medicaid have ceased being insurance policies for the elderly and the poor, respectively, long ago. They have become medical practice dictatorial federal programs to rule over the doctor-patient interaction. They have become mechanisms to take patient-care decision making out of the hands of the local medical doctors and take the Constitutionally-enshrined regulatory authority away from the states and bring it all under the control of the federal government.

The Art of American Health Care

Some commercial health insurance companies are apparently exempt from anti-collusion and anti-trust regulations and some of them collude with each other, or collude with Medicare, to model their policies and prices on Medicare policies and prices. Unless doctors and patients are willing to do cash-only business, then they are powerlessly subjected to this tyranny.

Contrary to popular belief, there is a private-entity, money-siphoning, middleman in the CMS relationship between the federal government and the participating medical doctors and participating hospitals. These are regional monopolies known as Medicare Administrative Contractors [MACs], they are for-profit contractors. They are responsible for processing medical doctor (Medicare part B) and hospital (Medicare part A) contracts and payments. It is often stated that they sometimes have a conflict of interest against doctors and hospitals.

Medicare part D is a disastrous Medicare-sponsored prescription drug payment plan that should have never existed. It must be discontinued.

Medical doctors via professional medical associations and state medical societies, along with hospital organizations go through annual proxy processes and CMS delegate meetings. Representatives from CMS supposedly hear from medical doctors and their various representative organizations along with hospitals and their various representative organizations about ways to improve the system, adjust payment policies, account for ICD codes and CPT codes, etc. A committee called the Specialty Society Relative Value Scale Update Committee [RUC] is formed to determine Relative Value Units [RVU] suggestions for CMS, supposedly to keep up with the value of medical doctor work.

RUC then makes formal, well-thought-out, supposedly unbiased, comprehensive recommendations to the policy makers at CMS. Then, each year in the October-November time frame, CMS holds private meetings and may ignore all the delegate's advice and the RUC's advice and even their own internal liaison's advice, and dictate protocols and prices which may harm doctors, private practices and patients, but which may benefit governmental budgets, government control over the health care system and big businesses.

Each year CMS comes out with numerous, arguably harmful, dictates like their recent disastrous programs including the Meaningful Use Program, the Pay for Performance Program, the Merit Based Incentive Payments System Program, the Alternative Payment Model Program, the Quality Payment Program, the Physician Quality Reports System Program, the Qualified Clinical Data Registry Program, the Delivery System Reform Program, the Medicare Payment Reform Program, the Medicare Access and CHIP Reauthorization Act and also annual drastic slashing of payments under the CPT system. CMS has even tried to resurrect the failed capitated-care construct of the 1990s under the new names of Accountable Care Organizations [ACO] and Medical Homes – these harmful programs pit the doctors against the patients. They pay a doctor or a health care organization which employs doctors a fixed annual fee. Money is spent on patient care out of this fixed annual budget and what is left over is retained by the health care organization and doctors. The less money spent on patient care, the more profit for the hospitals and doctors. The payer (for example, Medicare) loves it because they can plan an annual budget and never spend over budget. The problem is, the patients suffer. Nearly every time this has been tried, it has failed quickly, but CMS keeps trying to impose it.

Medical doctors, hospitals and health care organizations have to reconfigure themselves to whatever radical changes CMS imposes on the health care world each January – with warnings less than two months in advance. In years past it used to amount to only a few minor changes with a goal of bringing about larger reform over time. Currently it amounts to many dramatic changes to bring about instant reform. By the end of each calendar year, just when the medical community is finally settling in to the needlessly disruptive changes imposed earlier that year, CMS changes it all again in a broad-reaching drastic approach. This annual chaotic senseless disruption to the health care system, just because CMS can't make up its mind, because CMS keeps changing its mind, because CMS keeps experimenting in a rapid-cycling fashion with the health care system, is a manifestation of societal madness. We must pull the plug on CMS. It is thrashing around and desperate, but it inevitably needs to die before it takes all of us down with it.

The Veterans Health Administration [VHA] health care and hospital system, as a subsidiary of the Veterans Administration [VA], is a dysfunctional system that must be abandoned. Our veterans are relegated to what is arguably considered one of the worst health care organizations in the country. One solution is to have all active duty military and veterans be eligible to be treated at any private or public facility in America paid for by the US government or by a US government-paid high quality health care insurance policy. Tricare is an insurance policy, a low-quality plan modeled after Medicare, provided by a division of the Department of Defense, reserved for active duty military personnel and their dependents. It is discontinued upon discharge and the VHA system then takes over for the individual veteran. It is ironic that military individuals, either active duty or veterans, are offered near the lowest level of health care options in America. However, politicians are offered the highest quality health care options and in some cases this privilege extends for their lifetimes.

I changed my mind, don't do away with the VHA hospital system: use it for the politicians. Then use the politicians' platinum plans for all military personnel, active duty and veterans, for lifetime access – they deserve it more than anyone.

Chapter Fifteen:

Electronic Health Records

1. Electronic health records [EHRs] sometimes known as electronic medical records [EMRs] remain a controversial component of the health care system. These EHR systems might be beneficial in certain circumstances. However, they have been mandated by the federal government in nearly all circumstances without convincing proof of their being beneficial or safe. Consider that the VA medical system has been exclusively using a very high quality electronic medical records system for decades, but medical care in the VA system is considered by many to represent one of the lowest quality health care options available. Note that presence or absence of EHR has little or nothing to do with quality of health care.

2. The EHR mandates were provisions of the American Recovery and Reinvestment Act [ARRA] and the Health Information Technology for Economic and Clinical Health Act [HITECH] and to some extent part of the Patient Protection and Affordable Care Act [PPACA or ACA]. The EHR mandates were also incorporated into the Medicare payments incentives and penalties programs over recent years, and also incorporated into various state regulations. The purported purpose of EHR mandates was to improve quality and convenience of patient care for the doctor and the patient and to improve accuracy and efficiency and coordination of care. The more likely purpose is to make it easier for the federal government to control and regulate medical doctors and patients.

3. Most EHR systems have a practice management component which deals with coding and billing and the business of patient encounters.   They also have a scheduling component for organizing doctors' schedules. They also have a chart component for patient medical records. It would be reasonable if the health care world would allow doctors the free will to participate, or not, based on their own practices' and patients' needs and desires. The mandate of the doctors who don't want to use EHRs causes unintended loss of efficiency and quality. The mandate of the doctors who do want to use EHRs manipulates them into using the systems in ways they do not want to, and also causes unintended loss of efficiency and quality.

4. It is mandated that patients have access to their electronic records online. Some patients do not want their records put in an electronic database, and do not want their records accessible online. Patients apparently have no choice; however, there is no law prohibiting a patient from demanding that their doctor or hospital NOT post their data into the EHR. Patients, if they so desire, must put a written request into their doctor stating that they will not allow their doctor or hospital to post information into an electronic database or have that data available online.

5. Most EHRs are easily hackable, are not secure and contain more than just health information. They are popular targets for identity theft and other fraud activity. Also, why mandate a system that is completely dependent on the internet? Internet service is unreliable and unsecure in many geographic locations. Additionally, if you consider that the American health care system is an issue of national security, and our government is currently in the process of foolishly giving away control of the internet to international forces, then converting the American health care

system to an exclusively online system is unwise and dangerous because it enables a significant security vulnerability.

6.   Even though these systems are federal mandates, the individual doctors and hospitals must bear the startup and ongoing costs, with no potential to increase revenue as offset. This increases the cost of health care and diminishes the doctor's ability to provide quality of care. Additionally, EHR brands seem to be exempt from antitrust considerations as there are entire geographic regions now under the dominant control of one brand – this is harmful and dangerous to the American health care system.

7. Many doctors are forced to work with two or three or more EHR systems because they have multiple hospital affiliations and each affiliation uses a separate system. The mandates include a requirement that all of these EHR systems "talk" to each other, but the doctors are forced to use mandated products that don't do what they are mandated to do – and pay for it out of their own pockets.   Some affiliated hospitals threaten the doctors with disenrollment (which can cause the loss of insurance contracts and the loss of patients) if the doctors don't pay (inflated rates) for use of their system. Some hospitals may hold the doctor's medical record hostage or block the doctor entirely from the system, using access as a weapon against the doctor to force the doctor to cater to its will. Responsible doctors will not allow themselves to be dependent on a hospital-based system and will have an independent EHR system, if any. Currently, there are no standardized mechanisms for portability or archival access for when a doctor switches from one brand of EHR to another. How is it that all those patient records can be effectively and securely ported into the new system? How will the doctor maintain access

to all those old records if they can't be ported? No doubt there will be even more costs to the doctor involved. This is yet another mandated feature that the vendors are supposed to provide, but most don't.

8. The use of EHRs systems is intended to reduce medical errors, but the opposite is often true. Once an erroneous piece of information is put into such a system, it is often impossible to get it out. Furthermore, most of these systems are now what is called "shared" systems. This means that the EHR is not just for that doctor and that patient. The EHR is for every affiliated doctor and for every patient that is seen by any of those affiliated doctors. Any doctor or nurse or medical assistant or receptionist or even billing clerk can access and see every piece of medical and financial information on every patient in the system at any time. Since so many people are entering information regarding any particular patient, it is impossible for one doctor to maintain accuracy and integrity of the patient data – and yet it is the doctor who will be always held accountable for the data and data breaches – not necessarily the hospital that forces the system to be a shared system, not necessarily the vendor that designed and maintains the system and certainly not the government that mandated the system.

9. These systems diminish the doctor-patient interaction. Now doctors are sitting in front of a computer entering data during the patient encounter instead of looking at the patient paying attention to the problem at hand. Most EHRs also have a notification system that instantly notifies the doctor if there is some potential error or potentially harmful drug interaction, etc. However, the thresholds for such notifications is very low and the spectrum is very broad, so notifications may pop up nearly

continuously and so will ultimately go ignored. This concept of notifications tries to take away the doctor's responsibility to be thoughtful and thorough. Therefore it provides disruption not safety. The only solution is to allow doctors to decide if they want to use EHRs or not, and, if so, let the doctor have complete autonomy in deciding which brand and which features to use, free from hospital or governmental control, free from being forced into "shared" systems, and free from insurance or governmental or hospital payment penalties or incentives. Patients must demand to NOT have their data put into a "shared" system. They must demand that their doctors use a private system that only the doctor and his immediate staff can access, and if another doctor or person needs access, it must be by written permission from the patient as a one time allowance.

10. Sinister control is coming, and has been creeping in already. The federal government is a willing participant on the side of hospitals in the battle between hospitals and doctors. Medical care that takes place within hospitals gets paid through the Medicare part A program which pays generously and has annual increases mandated. Private practice community-based clinical medical doctors get paid through Medicare part B which may pay them less and less each year and which has been subject to annual governmental budget cuts. The federal government, through a dizzying number of ever changing and growing mandates and regulations, favors the hospitals since the hospitals have the ability to hire personnel to oversee all of this and manage it for their employed doctors. However, the independent doctors in the community ultimately won't be able to keep up. More and more doctors will be forced to cross over to the dark side of hospital employed positions. Once all the medical doctors are

employed by hospitals and there are no independent doctors left, then hospitals will believe they won the battle, but that is not the case. The hospitals will realize that they were just useful idiots for the federal government as the government will then implement a single payer government-run system. All hospitals and doctors and payments in the health care system will be 100% under the control of the federal government. States and private businesses will have little to no say in the system. The EHRs and the hospital conglomerates are the most expedient venues to enable this absolute governmental control to happen more quickly. The vendors of the EHR systems are also useful idiots for the federal government, which will allow them unbridled profits and all kinds of exemptions and forego any significant scrutiny, until it is all in place, then the profits will be gone and there will be only one government-run EHR for all citizens.

When a doctor enters data into an EHR, related to a patient encounter, currently there is substantial freedom regarding how he enters the information, what tests he orders through the system and what prescriptions he orders through the system. However, at some hospitals, the doctor cannot enter free-form text or dictate text. He must go through, in real time, with the patient present, clicking on options in drop-down boxes. If the options are not there, there might be ways to customize, but this will require special authorization and take a long time, even if approved. Then when the doctor gets to diagnostic test options, the option he wants may not be available, only the options the hospital or insurance plan wants him to choose will be possible. The same goes with treatment options, the proverbial blue pill and red pill problem. The doctor might know that the red pill is best, but the blue pill is cheaper – both pills are promoted to treat the same diagnosis, but the doctor knows that the blue pill doesn't work well, but, in his EHR, he will not be allowed to prescribe the red pill. This is already happening at the hospital level with employed, typically academic doctors, with hospitals motivated by reducing costs for the sake of profits. It will be a simple step for the government to take this over once they have driven all of the private practice, community-based, clinical medical doctors out of business.

Chapter Sixteen:

Electronical Health

I define "electronical health" as physical and mental health relative to electronic device exposure.

1. The phrase "smart phone" is popular. However, the smarter your phone is, the dumber you become. For improved brain health, development and longevity, rely on your brain more and your devices less.

2. Social media, as it is practiced today, is a form of slavery. While those individual users who engage in social media sites believe the sites are there for their use and benefit, it is really the other way around. The individual users are there for the site's use and benefit. In many cases, the user does most of the work, provides all of the content and actively solicits others to use the site. In many cases, the owners of a site can use and manipulate the data, secretly change the settings at random, "sell" or "rent" access to advertisers or others, censor the information, arbitrarily ban users and delete their content, engage in propaganda campaigns, share personal and private data with the government and often accept no liability for any consequences – even in cases of rape or death of users resulting from using the site. In such cases, the site owners then make all the profits while the ones that do most of the work and provide most of the content make nothing – seems like slavery.

3. The primary motivation for a user's participation in social media is narcissism and an obsession with microcelebrity status.

This is understandable with politicians, media personalities or sports personalities, who may have what is considered true celebrity status. Social media enables the common man to maintain the delusional belief he is worshiped – or allows the common man to worship himself. The use of social media can contribute to the development of mental illness, especially anxiety and depression. The obsessive use of social media cause people to squander their precious lives. Self-respecting people, reasonably intelligent people, people of healthful minds and of healthful spirits, avoid participating in social media. If you participate in social media, even if just occasionally, you are sacrificing a component of your mental and physical well-being. Any respectable business would be best to avoid engaging in social media as currently configured. Health care workers and medical doctors sometimes violate patient privacy and post inappropriate information. Any responsible health care worker or medical doctor would be best to avoid engaging in social media as currently configured.

4. Social media is one of the best tools that unsavory individuals can use to coordinate disruptive, anarchistic or otherwise criminal behavior. Even though social media venues enable and support criminal behavior, somehow, many social media companies and site owners seem to be given immunity regarding civil and criminal liability. If the granting of such immunity would end, then we would see an immediate reduction in criminal usage.

5. Social media is a great source of information for criminals to find naïve unsuspecting victims to perpetrate a broad spectrum of criminal acts including identity theft, rape, larceny, etc.

6. Social media is an effective venue for bullying, it will allow almost any bully to go so far as to induce suicide in its victim – imagine that, being able to get away with murder.

7. Social media is an effective venue to initiate adulterous affairs leading to the breakup of marriages and families.

8. Personal interaction with electronic screens, social media and electronic devices is addictive to the extent that serious health consequences arise such as sleep disturbance, attention distraction, poor posture, neck pain, finger joint injury, diminished intelligence, muscle deconditioning, sedentary lifestyle consequences, vision problems, brain developmental retardation, diminished motor function, diminished hand eye coordination, dysfunctional social development, psychological problems, and more. Personal interaction with social media and electronic devices results in untold costs to businesses due to lost productivity as workers are distracted all day long texting or updating and checking social media data. Personal interaction with social media and electronic devices results in classroom disruption and interferes with education.

9. People distracted by electronic devices, taking selfies, texting and the perpetual call to social media wind up causing car accidents or falling to their deaths. There is a common and traceable electronical death wake.

10. The internet, electronic devices, electronic games and social media provide the substance of such addictions that must be treated as a health liability no different from alcohol consumption or illicit drug use. Children are not smarter just because they are swiping screens at an early age – instead they are being robbed of irreplaceable time-limited opportunities of cognitive and

motor development. If you can't go for two days without access to a smart phone or computer device, then you are seriously ill. You must limit your exposure each day and take at least one day off (24 hours in a row) per week from electronic interaction (especially from anything with an electronic screen) in order to maintain minimal electronical health.

Since the trend toward increased use of electronic devices and social media is unlikely to reverse in the near future (it is the equivalent of the California gold rush of our day), then I encourage individual users to become more knowledgeable regarding personal health and personal safety. I encourage device makers, site owners and site developers to be mindful of these issues and develop the next generation of electronic devices and social media sites that respect people's privacy, cater to their safety, maintain their security, expunge criminal activity, ban violence, accept appropriate liability, share profits with users who provide content, and even provide appropriate health and safety warnings to users (similar to warnings for use of cigarettes or alcohol).

Chapter Seventeen:

Commentary on Selected Contemporary Health Topics and Societal Health Issues

1. Prevention of problems, to whatever extent possible, is the best way to maintain health – health of the individual, health of the community and health of the society. The old saying is true: "Choose your parents wisely." Genetics plays the single most important role in determining health. After that, the infinite environmental circumstances and influences exerted on individuals and on their community and on their society will have the greatest impact on health.

It is possible to optimize your genetic potential, but it is likewise possible to squander your genetic endowments based on environmental factors, based on your lifestyle choices and even based on choices society makes for you by its intervention in your environment and in your lifestyle. Consider a new saying: "Choose your country wisely, choose your state wisely." It is important to understand that all humans are NOT created equal, are NOT born into equivalent circumstances, and are NOT treated equally.

2. The conception of a child in the womb, destined for a viable birth, combining genetic material from the father and from the mother, with additional spontaneous mutations (as may occur with any natural conception), will result in a human that is

intended to be different and unique from every other human that has ever been born. Since humans are constantly moving geographically, since the environment is constantly changing, since the concept of community is constantly evolving and since the degree of societal intervention is constantly fluctuating, then this brilliant design feature built into the process of human procreation allows for the human race to continue to survive and to thrive.

3. Family, defined as a father and a mother together with their biological offspring, is, always was, and always will be, the immutable gold standard foundation building block of a healthy human society. There is no excuse for any society to try to tear it down as the ideal and standard with the excuse that it is difficult or even impossible for some people to achieve or to maintain. This statement has nothing to do with any religion, and must be understood within the context of human nature and the lessons learned throughout human history. It is difficult or impossible for some people to walk, and so should we eliminate walking for the sake of the few? No, but we must support those who cannot walk. A healthy society must protect and promote this family standard – or else death to such a society will occur. A kind and successful society will understand that when this gold standard is not met, for whatever reason, then alternative family structures will naturally arise to substitute. These alternatives must be thoughtfully woven into society, but not encouraged or promoted by society as being preferable.

The definition of marriage must be left to theologians and anthropologists, not legislators and judges. It is my personal and professional opinion that the U.S. Supreme Court decision which instituted government-sanctioned same-gender marriage, solely by the decree of five justices, was one of the darkest days in the history of the judicial branch of the United States of America. This was a situation whereby the decision was made based on the political feelings of the justices and not based on interpretation of the U.S. Constitution. This was a situation whereby the Justices acted as legislators. This was a situation of tyranny. If you consider that defining marriage is a religious act, then this constitutes our government's establishing specific government-sanctioned religious principles to the exclusion of all others. This has contributed to the ever-diminishing health of our American society. This has caused the citizenry to continue to lose faith in American government. This has pitted citizen against citizen. This has proven the recent and growing belief that American society is no longer protected by the rule of law and the U.S. Constitution, but is subject to manipulation by political parties and influential people.

There are no wise adults in charge in America at this time. There is little honesty or integrity. There are no statesmen. There are no honorable men and women. There are no leaders – only puppet rulers – in America today. I am not saying that I am for or against same-gender unions or marriage, it does not matter what any of us are for or against. People in America must be free to do what they desire as long as it does not harm others or prohibit others from their achieving their own desires. I am saying that the government must not be the entity that defines marriage. I say this for so many reasons, but mostly because if we let the government define marriage one way today, then it will have the authority to define marriage another way in the future – we must not give it that level of control over our lives.

A simple solution to that question before the Supreme Court could have been to rule that the United States government has no place in defining marriage aside from being allowed to ban polygamy due to its potential manifestation as slavery. Since the concept of spousal benefits was considered one of the motivations for litigation, then the legislature could legislate that the government can no longer provide spousal benefits of any kind. Spousal benefits could be converted to couple benefits. Every single adult citizen could then be entitled to designate one other adult as their coupled beneficiary. It could be a spouse, it could be a friend, it could be a neighbor and it could be changed at any time. The coupling would not have to be mutual. For example, a husband could list his wife as his coupled beneficiary, but the wife could list her sister as her coupled beneficiary. However, each citizen could not be beneficiary to more than one person. Therefore, in the above example, the wife could not then be the coupled beneficiary listed by her sister because she is already listed as the coupled beneficiary to her husband. Problem solved, government would be out of the marriage business, and all people would be treated equally, including single people who are still being treated unequally under the law in violation of their Constitutional rights.

4. Gender issues are of a medical and mental health nature and not of a legislative or civil rights nature. All children, even as young as two years old, are confused about their gender at some point in their upbringing, and some are confused for longer periods than others. This fact does not excuse the role of the parent from teaching and reinforcing gender in that child commensurate with genetics and genitalia (corresponding gender). Parents who are not teaching and reinforcing

corresponding gender, or who are not successful at teaching and reinforcing corresponding gender, whether willfully or not, are putting their child at tremendous risk for severe psychiatric issues in the future. In turn that will result in a high likelihood of a poor quality of life or even self-destructive behavior. Such parents need help. Furthermore, such children must not be used as pawns in social agenda or political propaganda warfare. In some rare cases it reflects mental illness of the parent. Of course, if the genetics are not simple male or female, or if the genitalia are not simple male or female, or if there is chimera involved (either in genitalia or brain tissue), then the parents must seek professional medical help to carefully and thoughtfully sort out the issue.

A note about chimera. The concept of chimera, as I am using here, refers to a fraternal twin of opposite gender whose entire body, at some point during fetal development, gets incorporated into the other twin's body. In some cases it may result in a microscopic cellular collection somewhere hidden in the body. What I am suggesting is that a portion of brain tissue or endocrine tissue could be a chimera and have an influence on the person's mind and body.

Gender reassignment surgery and hormonal treatments sometimes enable a person to more convincingly impersonate the opposite gender. Even though these procedures are lawfully practiced in the United States, they are being done without adequate research to designate clear indications or to fully assess outcomes. Unless there is an issue of an individual's genetics or genitalia not being simple male or female, then any doctor performing such interventions is engaging in a form of cosmetic dysmorphing surgery, albeit with patient consent. If such interventions are performed on children below the age of personal consent, in my professional opinion, then this constitutes child abuse. Any patient seeking such interventions is experiencing, potentially, a form of mental illness, a subset of body dysmorphic disorder or gender dysphoria. Such a patient, potentially, has a high risk of self-destruction, but that risk may increase if such a surgery is performed. These are issues for wise and experienced medical doctors, not for politicians and legislators.

Transgender issues are gaining media and legislative attention in recent years. A transgender individual is currently defined as an individual who "identifies" as being the gender opposite of what that individual's genetics dictate. This can occur in individuals just having fun psychologically messing with society. It can occur as a willful desire. It can occur as a peer-group or social media cult-like influence or it can occur as a manifestation of mental illness, as a subset of body dysmorphic disorder or gender dysphoria. Many such individuals need medical help, they do not need lawyers, politicians, legislators and judges to re-write the rules of society and reshape it to such an individual's current desire. Re-writing the traditional rules of American society will not help these individuals feel better or get better. However, society must reasonably accommodate such individuals. Accommodations must include access to unbiased medical and psychological care, and access to means to maintain privacy. It is appropriate to have gender-neutral, individual-use, public bathrooms, showers and locker rooms for such individuals or for ANY individual who desires or needs more privacy. It is a form of fascistic tyranny to force multiple genders to intermingle in public restrooms or shower rooms, against their will, especially if involving children, and extra especially if including children with adults – such a misguided attempt at assuaging the feelings of suspected or alleged transgendered individuals is being dictated by governmental actions in the form of "bathroom laws." The members of the "transgender community" are just willing pawns (if not anarchist activists), but will be eventual victims of this governmental intrusion. Are we now going to create a "gender-police force" to periodically investigate and "search" people?

Many complain that the "bathroom laws" in some states go too far by letting people choose to use multiple occupancy gender-specific bathrooms and locker rooms and shower rooms based on the gender they want to be in the moment, rather than based on their genetic gender. I say such laws are not necessary or do not go far enough. I say they are not necessary because transgender individuals have been discretely using the bathroom or locker room of their choice already and do not need a law for it. I say they do not go far enough because even though the stated purpose of such laws is to prevent discrimination against transgendered individuals, they do nothing to address a long list of other forms of discrimination or else they cause other forms of discrimination. Like most people in America today, I am against any form of discrimination. Such bathroom laws will discriminate against individuals who identify with each of several prominent religions that prohibit such comingling of genetic genders. Such bathroom laws will discriminate against individuals who identify with the absolute need for personal privacy in such circumstances. Such bathroom laws will discriminate against individuals who identify as disabled individuals who have an attendant of the opposite gender or of a different species. Such bathroom laws will discriminate against individuals who identify as having family needs of mixed genders, and so on.

My professional opinion is that true transgender individuals have chimera brain tissue of the opposite gender relative to their genitals and chromosomes (or vice versa). By legislating a politically motivated "solution" and forcing that on society, only chaos and anger (both overt and covert) will be brought to communities, not healing for the transgender individuals. Such ill-conceived actions will contribute to the diminishing health of society and may put people's health and life at further risk.

Furthermore, such bathroom laws will have unintended consequences. I can think of many, and I am sure there are many we will not see until later. As one example, think of prison life. If it is now considered, by politicians and governmental bodies, a form of civil rights violation to force an individual to be segregated away from the gender that individual identifies with, then many male prisoners will identify as women so they can be moved to the female block, have a female bunkmate and engage in "lesbian" sex.

I want readers from the future to understand that our American society is impotent, cowardly and leaderless in the year 2016. There are atrocious acts of genocide going on in parts of the Middle East, Africa and Asia – we are doing little about that. However, American federal, state and city governments are feverishly focused on micromanaging our public bathrooms and legislating what size soft drink we can order in a restaurant. Attention politicians: you should be ashamed of yourselves, step aside and let true leaders emerge.

The concept of legislating that a person can be what he identifies as, rather than what he is, amounts to government-sanctioned suspension of reality. I identify as having 20/20 vision, even though I am blind, and so it will be a violation of my civil rights to deny me a driver's license. I identify as being the owner of my neighbor's car so when I took it, it wasn't really theft, and I am innocent of any crime. If I am a male elite marathoner and I enter the Boston Marathon as a woman because I decide to identify as a woman, how is that fair? This amounts to government-sanctioned selfishness under the pretext of a medical necessity. This is a symptom of the feebling, gullibility, senility and mental illness of American society and of the current American government. Use your imagination: where will this litigated-sanctioned anarchy end, or else, where will it lead us?

Many people at this time are concerned about the potential for the following hypothetical news report becoming reality in the near future: "It was a great day for the civil rights movement. It harkens back to the historic days when blacks were finally allowed to share water fountains with white people, when women were allowed to vote, when gays and lesbians were allowed to marry the person they loved, when the transgendered were allowed to use the public shower of their choice, when bestiality was decriminalized and when protection of incest marriage was signed into law. Finally, after many years of legal wrangling, and after centuries of living in the shadows, the rights of pedophiles are now finally protected. In a six to five ruling, the Supreme Court has finally cleared the way for eliminating the age of consent and parental consent for sexual relations between adults and children. Charles Brownt, age 43 and his partner Justin, age seven, plaintiffs in the case, were seen celebrating outside the courthouse while Justin's parents were taken to a local hospital by ambulance because Justin's father suffered a heart attack minutes after the ruling was handed down..."

Privileges for special interest groups are not civil rights. The spirit of community-driven civil rights has been conquered by the demon of government-sanctioned civil anarchy.

The government must be evicted from our bedrooms, our bathrooms and our exam rooms.

Politicians must stop trying to "make history" and instead must learn from history. There is nothing new under the sun, including politicians being used as tools for oligarchs. It has all been done before, many times, in every way imaginable throughout past eons of civilizations. Politicians, lacking wisdom of human nature and willing to be used in exchange for money and fame, exhibit an ignorance of history. American civilization has come to be the way it is because of innumerable iterations by far wiser people of the past who have discovered what works best. Naive, buyable politicians of today use their positions of influence to manipulate society into reverting to a more primitive era (but call it progressive). They force us to re-experience why this or that societal construct is a big mistake. Society, and most individuals, will suffer, but those who bought the politicians will conquer and profit in the chaos.

5. Legalizing illicit drug use in the general population, as is currently being experimented with regarding marijuana in several states, is a dangerous experiment using American citizens and their children like laboratory rats. This provides no benefit to society (other than making a few insiders rich) and is definitively harmful to individuals, communities and American society. These are medical issues to be guided by medical doctors, not issues to be decided by politicians and legislators or controlled by popular vote. This sort of experiment has already occurred in certain segments of the American population and in large segments of

various human populations time and time again throughout
history throughout the world. It has always led to harm of the
individuals and diminishment or destruction of the society.
American society, and its leaders, must stop following or
repeating the path of doomed experiments.

Many people who are in jail today are in jail either directly
or indirectly due to the use of illicit drugs. Drug users need
medical doctors and treatment, not jail.

There is an opioid addiction crisis and an opioid-induced
death crisis in America today – medical doctors need to be leaders
involved in the solution. Medical doctors must not be in collusion
with politicians and businessmen to legalize and profit from
"recreational" drugs. "Medical-use marijuana" may have
legitimate medical applications; however, considerations
regarding appropriate indications, age restrictions, formulas and
dosing are still experimental.

6.   Contrary to popular belief, and contrary to frequent
advertisement, alcohol consumption has little to no proven net
health benefit when all health factors are considered together. It
is true that at certain times in human history, at certain locations
throughout the world, consuming an alcoholic beverage was safer
than drinking the local water, and led to a longer healthier life,
but that was when the average life span was 30 years old and
when we had limited understanding of toxins and infections.
Alcohol consumption will diminish cognitive performance, will
cause nutritional deficiencies, will lead to psychological problems,
can cause seizures, can cause neuropathy, can shorten lifespan,
can lead to intoxication, will impair motor function, will disrupt
college education and often leads to motor vehicle accidents

which often result in fatalities. There are almost no good reasons to consume alcohol, and there are no good reasons to become intoxicated. I am not advocating for prohibition, but alcohol is a drug with frequent deleterious effects. I am advocating that we, as a society, take this much more seriously. If it were to be brought up for FDA approval today, it would be considered a controlled substance requiring a special prescription by an appropriately qualified allopathic medical doctor and it would not be available over the counter. Death by alcohol, or death by drunk driver, is a huge serious problem in America today. It is not being appropriately addressed. More people are killed related to alcohol than from guns annually in America. One solution is to prohibit driving until 24 hours after there is any alcohol in the body. This must be explored in greater detail.

7. There are currently issues of "politically correct" speech, "micro-aggression" speech, "safe spaces" and "cry-bullies." In the United States of America, the Constitution and the Bill of Rights protect the freedom of speech of every citizen. Even though the federal or state governments may not be blocking this freedom, coordinated efforts sanctioned or paid for by political organizations, media organizations, social media companies, academic institutions, and the like are suppressing, shaming, penalizing, punishing, expunging or otherwise destroying freedom of speech and actively engaging in propaganda campaigns. I suspect the real reason is a bullying attempt by some organizations to gain influence to control peoples' thoughts in order to unnaturally reshape society for their exclusive benefit. This is not a philosophical movement. However, addressing the philosophical merits, American citizens must be allowed to say whatever they want without reprisal or arrest or lawsuit. Except,

statements of direct threat must still be subject to investigation and even prosecution. Additionally, American citizens must actively exercise their right to say whatever they want (except direct threats) so society can get used to it again. Decades ago, American citizens used to be able to say just about anything to anyone – there wasn't a misconceived expectation of a right, or entitlement, to not be offended as there is now. Remember, rights are powers you retain to protect yourself against your government, rights are not powers your government uses to protect you against your peers. If you don't like what a person says, grow a thicker skin and walk away. It's that simple; you and society will be healthier for it.

8. The failure of an individual to succeed in America is the individual's responsibility. No individual can blame someone else or blame American society for his own failure. If you blame your parents or your upbringing or your skin color or your finances or your neighbor or your gender or your religion or your ethnicity or unfairness or your height or your weight or whatever else for your failure, then blame is the source of your failure and you must learn to believe in yourself instead. If you think you need a law or a government program or an entitlement or some type of advantage or some other you-name-it condition in order to succeed, then dependency is the source of your failure and you must learn to believe in yourself instead. Whoever you are, if you believe in yourself, if you believe you can succeed and you work at it nonstop regardless of obstacles, then you will succeed!

9. American society currently ignores vulnerabilities that keep it in a crippled state. Attention to mental health – especially of children, of post-partum women and of young men – is at a barbaric status in this country. Attention to mental health as it

relates to violence, access to firearms and criminal-like behavior is at a barbaric status in this country. We need to increase the number of mental health doctors and clinicians by at least one hundred fold, and pay them double what they are making now, and increase the capacity of mental health care facilities by at least one hundred fold, just to begin to address the magnitude of the problem. Health insurance payers must recognize this need and allocate appropriate resources.

10. Strains and stresses on the individuals of our American society are magnified year after year, essentially institutionalized in our way of life. As a society we are not very humane with ourselves, but at the same time we have become too enabling of irresponsibility. There is a sleep deprivation crisis, there is an electronic overload crisis, there is a productivity-obsession crisis, there is a thought-and-speech-control crisis, there is a narcissism crisis, there is an entitlement crisis, there is a substance-dependency crisis, there is a sedentary crisis, there is a litigation crisis, and more.

Many Americans are addicted to benzodiazepines, amphetamines, opioids, alcohol, caffeine, "recreational drugs," tobacco, electronic devices, social media and entitlements. Some of these Americans do not seek substances, diversions and advantages because of pain, necessity or disability. They seek substances, diversions and advantages because they are irresponsible with ordinary consciousness and struggle to merely get through each day – otherwise they are made into addicts by those who wish to control them and profit from them.

Chapter Eighteen:

Sports Concussions

1. In recent years there has been misinformation propagated regarding sports concussions. Commensurately there has been an abundance of questionable products and services offered to profit from the fear and ignorance of unsuspecting victims (doctors and patients). This is a specific contemporary health topic and societal health issue that I choose to explore in greater detail. I do this in an attempt to counterbalance the overwhelming flow of misinformation being spread among athletes and even among medical doctors.

2. I propose defining concussion as comprising three parts:

First, it is a *mechanism of injury* whereby the brain is shaken or rotated relative to the skull. This may be achieved by a blow to the head, by rapid acceleration, by rapid deceleration, by rapid tumbling of the body or by rapid rotation of the head.

Second, it is a *neuropathophysiological process* that results from a concussive mechanism of injury. It is a process that results in a specific spectrum of abnormal brain function on a cellular and intracellular level. Nerve cells in the brain are often metaphorically represented as electronic devices (neuron cell bodies) that transmit electrical signals via wires (axons) to other nerve cells. In the case of concussion, it is more helpful to portray the neuron cell body as a factory and the axon as a collection of precisely coordinated conveyor belts carrying raw materials to the factory and carrying products away from the factory. When the brain is concussed, products temporarily cease being manufactured in the factory (neuron cell body) and the multiple conveyor belts stop moving or move more slowly or move in a disorganized fashion. The timing of delivery of finished products to the end of the axon is halted, slowed or mis-coordinated. The timing of delivery of raw materials to the neuron cell body is halted, slowed or mis-coordinated. Depending on the location within the brain where the nerve cells were concussed, that particular function or spectrum of functions will be disrupted.

Third, it is a *clinical syndrome* that results from a concussive mechanism of injury which has resulted in a neuropathophysiological process which has crossed a threshold of dysfunction to produce symptoms. (If the injury does not cross that threshold to produce symptoms, then the mechanism of injury is called "sub-concussive.") The concussion clinical syndrome may include one symptom or may include many symptoms or may include a series of changing symptoms. The clinical syndrome may last for a few minutes, a few hours, a few days, a few weeks or a few months. The clinical syndrome that results from the concussive mechanism of injury and pursuant neuropathophysiological process may give birth subsequently to one or more independent clinical disorders that might evolve and endure for weeks, months or years; continuing even after the concussional neuropathophysiological dysfunction has resolved.

The clinical symptoms will often depend on the specific region or regions of the brain that are concussed. The threshold for emergence of symptoms will depend on multiple factors including genetics, gender, training, pre-existing medical diagnoses, pre-head-trauma illness or pre-head-trauma injury, and many unknowns. The clinical symptoms can include dizziness, headache, vertigo or vestibular dysfunction, amnesia, impaired cognition, seizure, diminished motor control, gait impairment, visual dysfunction, altered hearing, altered emotions, bizarre behavior, tingling, nausea, vomiting, etc. Common disorders that may be born out of the concussion, and which may persist after the concussion has resolved, include headache disorder, sleep disorder, affective disorder (anxiety, depression, grief and panic), vestibular disorder, neuralgia and others. Of note, a concussion may or may not co-exist with other forms of traumatic head injury or traumatic brain injury, for example, skull fracture, subdural hematoma, etc.

3. By its medical definition, concussion is the mildest form of traumatic brain injury and results in complete resolution with no future consequences. However, the word mild refers to the relative magnitude and duration of brain damage. The symptomatology associated with a concussion may be dramatic and debilitating, and so must not be considered mild. Medical symptoms that persist beyond a few months usually represent one of the following: a brain injury other than concussion, a neuropathological process that was born out of the consequences of the concussion but has taken on a life of its own, a coincidental medical process unrelated to concussion, otherwise the patient may be pretending for the purpose of secondary gain. If litigation is involved, the symptoms notoriously persist, not necessarily due to the patient's pretending for the purpose of secondary gain, but due to one of the following: true fear that something bad and permanent has occurred, a strongly held belief that no one will believe the truth of what has happened unless symptoms are displayed, or getting poor and delayed care initially while pending authorizations for tests and treatment.

4.   There is no current standard of objective diagnosis.   The diagnosis is therefore made by the clinical judgment of the examining medical doctor based on context, history, symptoms, physical exam and the medical doctor's experience.   Currently, there is no test or technology which can definitively make the diagnosis.

5.   There are no universally effective medications to treat the symptoms of concussion, especially not in the acute phase (hours to days after the concussion).   Medications administered in the acute phase might produce unpredictable adverse side effects, therefore they are best withheld.   However, medication may be necessary considering other injuries which might have occurred at the same time as the concussion (for example, a brief course of opioid medication during recovery from surgery for fracture repair may be appropriate).   Medications that were prescribed prior to the concussion may need to be withheld due to potential for new adverse effect (for example, amphetamine-like substances).   Cognitive and physical rest for hours or days after a concussion may be appropriate, but rest for weeks or months, under any circumstances, is harmful.

In recent years, perpetual cognitive and physical rest has been promoted by medical doctors and other health care clinicians, based on faulty theories and inexperience.   This has led to the emergence of some of the most difficult to treat cases. Concussed patients who have been instructed to rest for weeks and months and in some cases years have the greatest challenge with reintegration back into normal life, work, education and sports activity – all unnecessary – all caused by the ignorant instructions and not caused by the concussion.

Sports Concussions

Some medical doctors recommend a limit to the number of concussions after which a student athlete should be barred from sports participation. Some say seven, some say three, but it is subjective and based on opinion not fact. Some of these medical doctors have loud voices and have had access to political ears and so then legislation often (inappropriately) follows. Some medical doctors focus their efforts on never clearing athletes to return to their sport, mostly due to the doctor's (unreasonable) fear and that it "seems to be" the safest decision to "protect" the athlete.

In my professional opinion, it is the role of the medical doctor to help the athlete get back to his sport and provide education regarding health issues. It is not the role of the medical doctor to ban the sport and try to (with a superiority complex) save the athlete from himself. Sports like American football, ice hockey, rugby, rodeo, boxing and mixed martial arts must not be banned, instead, the athletes must be provided with informed consent to the known and suspected risks and be provided with effective strategies of protection and recovery. We allow young men and women to volunteer as soldiers for combat duty (in the past the men were drafted), and we do not ban combat duty due to its risk of physical harm and death. So why should we prohibit other men and women from choosing to voluntarily participate in sports which may have a risk of harm or even death? In some cases these athletes are paid at astronomically higher rates of compensation than those in the military. Consider that car accidents, use of recreational drugs, use of alcohol, gun violence and opioid prescriptions each lead to greater rates of morbidity and mortality annually than sports concussions, but we don't think of banning such access.

The most useful decision-making information regarding future sports participation of an athlete regarding concussions is the following: Consider the ease with which the athlete gets a concussion in that setting, and the magnitude and duration of concussion symptoms. If the threshold is low and the symptoms are great with long duration, then consider switching sports.

6. There are many questionable products and services currently marketed for prevention, treatment and assessment of concussion. Opportunists have marketed magic helmets, magic head bands, magic chin straps, magic mouth guards, magic eye wear, magic electronic devices, magic apps, etc., touted to prevent the incidence of concussion, to assess the effects of concussion or to accelerate recovery. There is no such magic device that will prevent concussion mechanism of injury, that will prevent pursuant neuropathophysiological response or that will accurately assess or diminish the pursuant clinical syndrome – that we know of yet. Helmets mostly protect against other types of head injury such as scalp lacerations and skull fractures. Ironically, helmets may increase the incidence of concussion because a player that wears a helmet may gain a false sense of security and so neglect to protect his head or else use his head as a weapon. All helmeted athletes must play as if they are not wearing helmets – they will then protect their heads more and minimize concussion occurrence.

7. There are many questionable products and services currently marketed for diagnosis of concussion. Computer-based cognitive testing, especially when administered by a non-neurologist or a non-neuropsychologist, is not a valid or reliable modality for diagnosing concussion or for assessing recovery from concussion or for assessing clearance for return to play [RTP].

Sports Concussions

Note: a valid test is one that accurately tests for the objective it is intended to test for. A reliable test is one that yields predictably reproducible results, regardless of any extenuating circumstances. As an example, a CT scan of the brain is valid for diagnosing a subdural hematoma – there will be no mistake. That same CT scan of the brain is also reliable for diagnosing a subdural hematoma. It is correct when the patient is conscious or unconscious, it is correct when the patient is drunk or sober, it is correct when the patient tries to fake symptoms or not, it is correct when the patient has to go to the bathroom or not, and so on. It will always show the subdural hematoma. The same cannot be said for computer-based cognitive testing. Such tests can "diagnose" a concussion when there is none, and they can miss the "diagnosis" of concussion when there is one. They can give differing results even under the same conditions, and the tester can fake, manipulate or "game" the results.

The concept of requiring cognitive testing as a "baseline" is a myth that may be perpetuated due to conflict of interest in the pursuit of financial gain on the part of those selling such tests or due to ignorance on the part of medical doctors utilizing such tests. There is no brand of cognitive test that is FDA approved for diagnosing concussion or assessing baseline against future concussion or assessing recovery for return to play after concussion – and yet this is how some people (inappropriately) use these tests. The concept of lack of validity and lack of reliability and non FDA approval can be expanded to evaluate various other electronic-based "diagnostic tools" such as smart phone apps, etc.

The Art of American Health Care

The following is an important message to professional sports organizations, school athletic programs and governmental agencies, consider yourself hereby warned:

It is important that professional sports organizations and school athletic programs recognize that administering a computer-based cognitive test as a baseline (or annually as refresher baselines) and then once or more after a concussion, for all of their athletes, does NOT constitute a concussion management program. We know that these tests arguably lack validity and arguably lack reliability (in spite of marketing hype) for diagnosing concussion. We know that, even though some of these products may be "FDA approved" as testing devices, they are NOT FDA approved for diagnosing concussion or for guiding concussion treatment or for determining fitness (or lack of fitness) for return to play. Since we know that such tests are being used by such organizations and programs for diagnosing concussion and for making return to play determinations, then that puts such organizations and programs at risk for liability because they DO KNOW that it is inappropriate, but they still do it. In cases where taxpayer funds are being spent, this constitutes a breach of governmental fiduciary responsibility.

The best objective measure we have at this time (although still inadequate) is baseline imaging to include brain MRI with diffusion tensor imaging, susceptibility sequences and quantitative volumetric analysis compared to age-matched (and perhaps gender matched) controls. This must be followed by post-head-trauma imaging with the same sequences. This can then be followed longitudinally over time at appropriate intervals. An additional objective measure is baseline and then serial electroencephalogram recordings.

In my practice, I find that formal cognitive testing (either computer-based or pen-paper-based), beyond a medical doctor's in-office routine mental status evaluation, is almost never needed in cases of concussion, and has NO IMPACT on the outcome of the patient. Formal cognitive testing, by a duly trained neuropsychologist, might be appropriate, at the discretion of the treating medical doctor, if there is a greater level of brain injury or if there is a superimposed cognitive or behavioral disorder unrelated to concussion.

8. When concussion mechanism of head injury occurs, the most important question is if the brain injury exhibits more than just concussional neuropathophysiology. That is what medical doctors need to explore at the time of concussion.

As medical doctors, we have identified brain injury sub-diagnoses such as brain contusion, intraparenchymal hemorrhage, microhemorrhaging, subdural hematoma, subarachnoid bleed, diffuse or focal axonal injury, disruption of brain organ autoregulation, malignant intracranial hypertension, etc., but there are definitely other types of brain injury sub-diagnoses that medical science has not yet discovered. It may be reasonable to leave the definition of concussion where it is, but I propose adding new brain injury sub-diagnoses: traumatic axonal microtubulosis or microtubulitis, traumatic neuronal membranosis or mebranitis, traction-induced neurotransmitter receptor erosion, shear-induced dendritic disconnection, and more. These new sub-diagnoses must be considered in acute, subacute, chronic and co-morbid manifestations. It is likely that technological advances in imaging modalities will eventually result in valid and reliable diagnostic biomarkers applicable to concussions as well as to these new sub-diagnoses.

There are some important practical considerations which are often neglected when considering consequences of concussions in humans: First, if you bang something hard enough or repeatedly, then it will get damaged. Second, some brains are more fragile than others: some athletes have "glass brains," and some athletes have brains that can be hit hard and repetitively with no consequences. Third, youthful brains are less susceptible to long term consequences of mild traumatic brain injury because of their greater plasticity compared to adult brains, so young children may benefit from very rough play in order to shake out the weak brain connections such that only strong connections remain.

9. "Concussion laws" have been legislated in every state, but were inspired by injuries that were not necessarily concussions. Each state law is merely a collection of opinions made into rules dictated to the citizenry. This amounts to legislators practicing medicine without appropriate training or licensing. Every "concussion law" or statute or regulation of every state needs to be nullified, and these issues need to be left up to experienced treating medical doctors working with their communities and their patient athletes on a case by case basis.

10. As inferred above, traumatic brain injury may lead to various chronic consequences; however, concussions are NOT KNOWN to cause Chronic Traumatic Encephalopathy [CTE]. It is extremely important to note that if a person suffers chronic consequences after a concussion, then it does not mean that person has CTE. CTE was formerly known as Dementia Pugilistica, and it has been described by other names. Some medical doctors and researchers state that there is a cause and effect relationship. They state that multiple concussions or multiple sub-concussive

events will lead to the condition that is currently designated as CTE. They might be correct; however, this cause and effect relationship is unknowable at this time. There have been no prospective case-controlled studies to prove this cause and effect relationship. There have been some case series published that provide anecdotal evidence of an association between the occurrence of CTE in athletes who have participated in contact or collision sports and who have experienced concussions – but that does not constitute a cause and effect relationship between CTE and concussions.

The vast majority of individuals with known repetitive head trauma do not wind up with CTE. CTE has been found in individuals with no significant history of concussion. CTE is almost unheard of in females even though females are known to be more susceptible to concussions than males. I suspect body blows, through a similar mechanism to blast injury in soldiers, may play a role. As the body is hit, the arterial system is compressed and brief acute spikes of blood pressure are conveyed to the brain. The cumulative effect of thousands of such incidences in an athlete may ultimately result in brain perivascular deleterious consequences – perhaps CTE – even without concussions.

"The fear of CTE" is a phenomenon I designate as a new clinical entity. It is challenging to treat. Many health care providers mistakenly inform concussed athletes that they are at high risk of developing CTE and inappropriately instruct athletes to discontinue sports participation. This often results in paralyzing fear, anxiety, depression, grief and panic in the patient athlete and in the family.

I propose that the phrase Chronic Traumatic Encephalopathy [CTE] be abandoned and the phrase Brain

Perivascular Phosphorylated Tauopathy or simply Brain Perivascular Tauopathy [BPT] take its place. This new phrase is more descriptive of the known brain pathology in such cases. BPT may be considered a subcategory of Tauopathy. There are other well-known subcategories of Tauopathy, some with known genetic defects. Individuals with BPT may exhibit clinical abnormalities (in the realms of behavioral, cognitive or physical) or may appear normal. Cases of BPT may progress rapidly or slowly. There may be a head-trauma association; however, the head-trauma may not necessarily cause BPT, instead, individuals with pre-existing BPT may be attracted to violence and hence wind up more likely experiencing head-trauma. Body blows which cause arterial-conveyed spikes of brain blood pressure may play a role. BPT is most likely something people are born with as a genetic pre-disposition (but we don't know what the genetic issues are yet). These people are more likely to be depressed, exhibit cognitive impairment, exhibit irrational behavior, exhibit criminal behavior and most often seek out contact sports as an outlet for their violent tendencies. If we take away that outlet, they may be more likely to become homicidal or suicidal even earlier; and so banning contact sports is not an appropriate option.

Every professional athlete involved in violent contact sports, such as American football, ice hockey, rugby, rodeo, boxing, mixed martial arts, etc., that faces the end of their active career, will face depression, idleness, financial issues and social issues. They will no longer get heightened media attention or a lucrative paycheck. They will experience physical deterioration as a consequence of aging and years of wear and tear in the sport. They will need appropriate counseling, education and guidance to make this transition healthfully. Many of these athletes turn to illicit drugs or alcohol and hence introduce an additional level of health risk. Those with BPT are at greatest risk, but preventing them from having been involved in contact sports in the first place may not be a viable solution.

There are rumors to the effect that professional sports team owners or leaders knew, many years ago, that concussions cause CTE (or BPT as I am calling it herein). How can that be when the greatest experts alive today still do not know this?

In considering CTE or BPT, there is ongoing research into methods of diagnosing the disorder prior to death and autopsy. There is no way to diagnose this condition in a living person at this time, and so there is no way to treat it directly. However, I propose that substances in the realm of tyrosine kinase inhibitors and NMDA receptor blockers be investigated as a potential treatments in those who are suspected of having it. If monitored appropriately, these types of treatments should be safe, and might be effective to control the symptoms and possibly even reverse the damage.

Chapter Nineteen:

The Art of Health Care

1. What is a health care system? Fundamentally, it is a system whereby appropriately trained and licensed allopathic medical doctors, as physicians and surgeons, care for people (patients) who are experiencing physical or mental illness, injury or degeneration. The best health care system will also include care in the form of preservation of health along with prevention of illness, injury and degeneration. All other involved people, facilities, equipment, technology, science, research, products, financial intermediaries, governmental bodies, regulatory agencies, community leadership, and constructs of societal mores and professional ethics are intended to assist and support the allopathic medical doctors' leadership role in caring for the patients. Whenever any person or group or agency or institution gains a preferential position inserted between the medical doctor and the patient, then the health care system becomes dysfunctional proportional to the degree of that outside intrusion.

The American health care system is in ruins. It is barely functional in some places and completely dysfunctional in others. The American health care system had been evolving over the course of centuries before the academic establishment, commercial entities and governmental forces invaded to overthrow its greatness.

The Art of Health Care

It is time for the American health care revolution. It is time for a renaissance of the once great American health care system. It is time for American medical doctors and American patients to take back the American health care system and build a wall against any future invasion by the academic establishment, commercial entities and governmental forces.

As we consider rebuilding this system, we must go back to the roots of how it emerged as the great system it once was. We must understand the destructive forces that culminated in its ruin. We must return to the focus of preserving and protecting the doctor-patient relationship as its immutable, priority, core principle. All other aspects of the new American health care system must then be secondary and tertiary revolving around this core principle.

2. Medical doctors must work as priority for their patients, not for their business employer, not for their hospital, not for their government, not for their academic title, not for the sake of purity to their personally chosen "specialty," not for their research project and not for the dictates of some insurance company policy. Medical doctors must shift their focus away from such distractions and seek innovative approaches to succeed at helping their patients heal and remain healthy. Medical doctors must be useful to their patients, help solve problems, not merely provide micro-suggestions or perform procedures which wind up being useless. Medical doctors must learn successful business and lobbying strategies. Medical doctors must lead the return to free market doctor-patient financial interaction.

Medical doctors must grow a new mindset whereby they do not shy away from being bold and demanding when interacting with governmental agencies, insurance company representatives, hospital administrators, academic institutional hierarchies, alternative practitioner organizations and even their own professional organizations if it is in the best interest of their patients. Many such representatives, administrators, institutions, practitioners and organizations have had no qualms about being increasingly bold and demanding of medical doctors over recent decades, primarily for their own inappropriate gain and not at all for the benefit of the patients.

3.   Patients must be guided by more efficient, timely, comprehensive and effective medical doctor encounters. They must receive counseling, education and more successful diagnostic and treatment strategies through their medical doctor encounters.   Patient satisfaction and favorable health care outcomes must increase. Health care costs to the patient must decrease, or at least be of greater value relative to the care received.   Patients must be protected against alternative practitioners deceptively engaging in allopathic medical interventions. Patients must be protected against the conflicts of interest inherent in the intrusions of governmental agencies, hospital administrators, academic departments, research programs, insurance companies, pharmaceutical companies, biomedical technology companies and otherwise commercial and institutional influence over the American health care system.

4. Governmental bodies must withdraw from paying for health care, must discontinue overly regulating health care and must completely abandon interfering with the doctor-patient relationship regarding diagnosis and treatment of medical and surgical issues. Governmental bodies must contribute toward individuals' funding of their own commercial health care insurance coverage; there must be universal coverage.

Governmental bodies must radically simplify the number and complexity of health care related agencies and drastically reduce the number of people they employ in such efforts. The federal, state, regional and local governmental bodies must still play roles in protecting the citizenry in the form of continuing certain agencies such as the CDC, the FDA, the departments of children and families, the medical examiner's offices, the states' boards of medicine, etc., but there must be tight and frequent oversight and review by an independent panel of clinical medical doctors which must have the authority to expand, reduce or even eliminate the role of such agencies based on appropriate core principles. The federal government must discontinue operating any and all facilities for active duty or retired military personnel and instead entitle complete freedom of active duty and veterans to access health care in the private practice setting, perhaps except in war zones, but even that could be privatized.

5.   Medical colleges and universities must dismantle their academic hierarchies related to the clinical practice of medicine and abandon the failed, biased, conflicted and innovation-inhibiting constructs of departments, divisions, chairs, endowed chairs, chiefs, professors, internships, residencies and fellowship programs.   There is no place for academia in the practice of modern clinical medicine and surgery. The system of academic medical doctors' attempting to practice clinical medicine has been tried for many decades and has turned out to be a dismal failure. This system of turning over control of clinical patient care to academia has become a commonplace experiment in many regions across America.   However, it is a system that blocks innovation, diminishes excellence, blocks competition, blocks free market forces, establishes conflicts of interest against

increasing quality of patient care and destructively enshrines failed academic medical doctors into positions of control and influence. Medical colleges and universities must be involved in providing initial basic education to medical students but then leave the students to be trained as clinical medical doctors and surgeons in apprenticeship positions working with experienced clinical medical doctor mentors in the community.

6. Licensing and certifying bodies must allow for fast and easy medical licensing reciprocity from state to state, especially concerning underserved geographic areas; it should take days, not months or years. Licensing and certifying bodies must establish a reasonable process for expediting unrestricted transition of medical doctors' authority between clinical specialties or at least for allowing broadening of medical doctors' spectrum of clinical authority, especially concerning underserved specialty needs. Today this concept is essentially impossible, or in the rare cases where it is achievable, it is complicated, costly, will require a series of extraordinary permissions from multiple authorities and will take five years or more, never with a guarantee of ultimate success. It must be a process available to any and all medical doctors, even including transitions from non-surgical to surgical and vice versa, and must be achievable within one year.

7. Commercial health care insurance companies must deal directly with the patients and not at all with the medical doctors or hospitals. The concept of using a pre-tax health savings account [HSA] or a flex spending account [FSA] must be expanded for the benefit of patients to be able to cover such costs prior to receiving reimbursements from insurance. Insurance reimbursements to the patients can then go back into these

accounts, with no tax consequences, once received. Commercial health care insurance companies must focus on supporting the doctor-patient relationship as a priority and be judged by patient satisfaction. There can be rating agencies that accumulate and publish data regarding the performance of such companies, and so patients can switch away from the bad ones to the good ones quickly and easily. Such companies must never interfere with the doctor-patient relationship regarding diagnosis and treatment of medical or surgical issues otherwise face crippling fines and penalties. Such companies must cover expenses for medical care across state lines and abandon the concept of "physicians in network." Such companies must process reimbursements to patients rapidly through a simple process without inappropriate denials and delays or otherwise face crippling fines and penalties. If there are concerns about high costs of insurance to the elderly or to the chronically ill, then the solutions will be in the free market combined with minimally invasive state regulations, not in the federal government. Furthermore, health insurance policies must not be limited to annual policies, and could be made multi-year term, or life-long, similar to life insurance policies.

8. Hospitals, medical centers and health care delivery-related organizations must abandon the practice of employing medical doctors, and must be owned by medical doctors. They must return to the system of the past whereby all medical doctors, as physicians and surgeons, were independent contractors and the hospital facility was merely a support-staffed-venue wherein the doctors and patients could safely engage in appropriate health care encounters of emergency care, critical care and surgical intervention. Such facilities' administrators must never interfere with the doctor-patient relationship regarding diagnosis and

treatment of medical or surgical issues otherwise face crippling fines and penalties. Large conglomerate hospital mini monopolies need to be busted up, and certificate of need regulations must be abolished in states that still have such regulations. New entities must have no barriers to compete with the well-established facilities: this will accelerate innovation, increase choices and drive prices down.

9. There must be no concept of medical malpractice litigation or medical product litigation against medical doctors, hospitals, pharmaceutical companies or biomedical technology companies. In its place must arise an equitable system of no fault insurance financed by recurring fees to medical doctors, hospitals, pharmaceutical companies and biomedical technology companies. Patients who are harmed in the health care system must have expedited access (days to weeks, not years) to appropriate financial compensation to support subsequent ongoing medical needs. Such a system must not exempt medical doctors, hospitals, pharmaceutical companies and biomedical technology companies from civil or criminal liability regarding fraud or criminal activity.

10. In this scenario, due to the emergence of a new medical free market economy, medical doctors, hospitals, pharmaceutical companies and biomedical technology companies must reconfigure their financial structures to reduce costs to patients. They will be forced to figure out new strategies for efficiency and success. All persons, entities and policies in the American health care system must be recalibrated to focus on the doctor-patient relationship as an absolute, immutable, sacred priority. Any person, entity or policy that violates this sacred priority must be banned from the American health care system of the future.

The Art of Health Care

It is only through adopting the foregoing principles that we will be able to make the American health care system great again.

Chapter Twenty:

The Ghost of American Health Care Past

1. Many decades ago medical doctors dedicated many years of their early lives, often in impoverished conditions, often living inside hospitals for years (hence the phrase "resident doctor"), often staying awake for days in a row, often putting themselves at serious risk of harm, all for the sake of becoming experts in the practice of clinical medicine or surgery.

2. Upon completion of medical school and internship and residency, medical doctors from decades ago became indisputable experts dedicated to the clinical practice of medicine and surgery in the pursuit of excellence.

3. The physicians and surgeons of this era were so dedicated and busy taking care of people that they had little time, or interest, in pursuing legislative issues or legal issues or regulatory issues or any issues outside of improving their excellence in the practice of the art of medicine and surgery – and there was usually little need for them to do so.

4. The physicians and surgeons of this era were appropriately respected and appreciated for their indispensable contribution to society, and, more than money, these medical doctors valued their role in society and received their greatest satisfaction from helping others.

5. The physicians and surgeons of this era wisely understood the balance of financial compensation: Wealthy people paid full price, ordinary income people paid a lower price, farmers paid with agricultural products, tradesman paid by performing a service, and those in poverty got free care. The medical doctor balanced his practice with a cross section of patients in such a way to remain financially solvent. They weren't great businessmen, but they didn't need to be, they were good enough at business management because medical business was fairly simple.

6. At that time it was understood that medical doctors were only human and the art of the practice of medicine or surgery was not an exact science, and doctors were not infallible machines, and doctors did not cause illnesses or injuries, and doctors did not make the dysfunctional lifestyle decisions that often caused patients to become chronically ill, and doctors did not decide the genetic disposition of the patients, and doctors did not control the patients' compliance with treatments, and doctors had no control over the limits of medical knowledge or technology. And so doctors were not liable for the outcomes unless there was fraud or criminal activity perpetrated. Although, there have been times in history when the doctor's life was held in the balance against the outcome of the patient – especially if the patient was royalty or some similar oppressively coerced situation.

7. Medical doctors of this era maintained an adversarial relationship with hospitals and health care organizations – understanding that they themselves were the ultimate advocates for what was best for the patient and for themselves, and understanding that the hospitals and health care organizations focused primarily on financial health over patient health. They were independent practitioners or in a private group practice, but

almost never would they allow themselves to be employees of the hospital or health care organization due to the serious conflict of interest that would then be set up.

8. Medical doctors of this era were dedicated to the extent that most aspects of their personal life would suffer to support their vocation – their calling – as a physician or surgeon. They were disturbed at all hours of the night or day, any day of the week, any time of the year, regardless of their own personal health or safety, regardless of family or friends or personal interests, in order to go out and take care of patients in need. During this era, each medical student, intern and resident went all out with mindboggling service for many years, in a survival of the fittest trial of endurance. Those that made it were so incredibly well trained and immune to sickness or fatigue or injury or psychopathology that they were essentially naturally selected to be the stalwart medical doctor physicians and surgeons of their future. They could be relied upon for all things at all times – even during the ravages of wartime. Those that didn't make it were not fit to be medical doctors and were dismissed.

9. Medical doctors of this era played leadership roles in their communities and their communities wisely included the medical doctors in efforts to improve and maintain community health.

10. Medical doctors of this era understood that the practice of medicine and surgery was an art that required a mature and wise understanding of human nature superimposed on the application of scientific knowledge and technology. The outcome had just as much to do with the way the doctor interacted with the patient and the patient's family as it did with identifying the correct diagnosis or prescribing the correct medication or performing the appropriate surgical procedure. It was understood that the

human body had the inherent ability to heal itself, and the doctor was there to facilitate that natural healing process.

Chapter Twenty One:

The Ghost of American Health Care Present

1. Currently medical doctors dedicate many years of their early lives, often in impoverished conditions, often living inside hospitals for days during their residency program, often staying awake overnight, often sacrificing personal leisure pursuits, all for the sake of achieving credentialing as a medical doctor.

2. Upon completion of medical school and internship and residency, medical doctors of today are sometimes considered experts in the clinical practice of medicine and surgery; however, they sometimes pursue teaching, research and publication distractions with the goal of climbing the academic professorship track and with the goal of achieving fame within the medical community.

3. The physicians and surgeons of today are rarely dedicated to taking care of people, because that is considered beneath their intelligence level, work best reserved for trainees and "physician extenders" such as residents, nurse practitioners and physician assistants. Many have no time, or interest, in pursuing legislative issues or legal issues or regulatory issues or any issue outside of self-promoting their academic climb or publications or speaking engagements. This has led to poorer patient outcomes, relative to available scientific knowledge and technology. This has led to legislative successes by a myriad of lobbying forces which have succeeded in undermining medical doctors' authority and

autonomy – to the extent that medical doctors have become merely algorithm implementers to be rewarded when they follow the algorithms and punished when they don't – and these algorithms are often conceived by groups of people and organizations that may not even include medical doctors – algorithms that focus on issues such as cost, tracking, reporting, coding, billing, monitoring, and ultimately controlling and manipulating patients and doctors. It has been legislated or litigated or otherwise allowed that non-medical-doctors can substitute for medical doctors – so this has inappropriately (and dangerously) given rise to the ever-encroaching expanded scope of the practice of nurses, physical therapists, psychologists, pharmacists, herbalists, nutritionists, naturopaths, homeopaths, chiropractors, massage therapist, acupuncturists, etc., into the actual practice of allopathic medicine.

4. The physicians and surgeons of today are almost universally disrespected and unappreciated for their work even when they do make substantial contributions to society or to an individual's life – they are considered no more than servants and their service is considered an entitlement. Medical doctors of today are often concerned about money because the cost of their many years of training has gone up exponentially relative to their ability to pay their debt through insurance reimbursements and income. The value of doctors' take home pay has gone down substantially every year for at least the past 20 years. This has caused doctors to increase their volume of patients and decrease their time with each patient and increase the spectrum of services provided based on billing potential, not necessarily based on patient need – just to be able to pay their bills. Doctors are not considered "rich" anymore. It is now rare to find a seasoned medical doctor

that is not burned out. Medical doctors of today are trying to retire earlier than the doctors of past generations, or at least switch to another career if they can. This significantly reduces their years of service and contributes to the worsening of the medical doctor shortage crisis. It is now rare to find medical doctors that still receive their greatest satisfaction from helping others.

5. The physicians and surgeons of today are mostly detached from understanding the balance of financial compensation because they rarely deal directly with the patient or the payer in this regard. Most are now in hospital or governmental employment positions working on a salary. The ever diminishing number of ones that remain in private practice deal almost exclusively with insurance companies and payment contracts. They have little or no power to fairly negotiate such contracts and so insurance companies (both commercial and governmental) essentially dictate what a doctor receives. The doctor is further constrained by federal and state laws regarding billing and collection issues. Some insurance companies are apparently immune to collusion and price-fixing which can take advantage of medical doctors, but medical doctors are essentially prohibited to engage in collective bargaining and are prohibited from going on strike. It is important for readers to understand that the fee that a medical doctor collects from a patient encounter is not his income. Out of that amount he has to pay his rent, his staff, his supplies, his utilities, his malpractice insurance, his taxes, etc., such that these days there is little left over for income. In many states, municipal workers such as toll-takers, sanitation workers, train-system employees, etc., can make more than medical

doctors in annual take home salary, and typically have superior retirement plans as well.

6. At this time it is expected that medical doctors are inhuman perfected machines due to the rumors of high quality medical training promulgated at academic facilities, and that the practices of medicine and surgery are exact sciences, and that doctors are somehow responsible for patients' illnesses or injuries, and that doctors are responsible for the dysfunctional lifestyle decisions that often cause patients to become chronically ill, and that doctors are responsible for the genetic disposition of the patients, and that doctors somehow control patients' compliance with treatments and that doctors have full access to unlimited medical knowledge and technology. The trend is toward making doctors liable for patients' outcomes under all circumstances. In some states, in some cases, trial lawyers can sue the doctor, the nurse, the receptionist, the housekeeping staff, the medical students, the residents, the building manager, the hospital, the practice manager and essentially anyone who has come into contact with the patient with the sole intent of making the litigation process so painful and complicated that everyone will just give up and give money. The majority of malpractice cases may be considered frivolous and unwarranted. Malpractice cases may result in windfall profits for the lawyer and law firm, sometimes the patient claimant will wind up with much less than the lawyers. Each and every malpractice suit that is brought against any medical doctor will remain as a permanent blemish on his record – even if he is proven completely innocent. There are no such consequences for the lawyers even if they lose. This sort of thing occurs even though the doctor is constrained from ordering tests and deciding treatments based on the "prior authorization"

concept whereby the patient's insurance company – not even other doctors – makes the ultimate decision about which tests a medical doctor can or cannot order and about which medication or treatments a medical doctor can or cannot order. Hospital-employed doctors likewise cannot make independent decisions, often the hospital sets algorithms, guidelines and protocols based on what is best for the hospital finances or due to some committee decision.

7. Medical doctors of today are increasingly less-well trained, less intelligent, less independent, have no business experience or financial expertise, and are chosen due to their disposition to obey and to not talk back. They tend to embrace their employed relationship with hospitals and health care organizations so they can have a guaranteed fixed income, predictable work schedule and be free to plan and frequently pursue personal and leisure activities. They defer to the hospital or health care organization to employ patient advocates. They consider that the focus of their work is for the benefit of the hospital or health care organization that employs them or else they consider that the focus of their work is to pursue research or academic professorship or fame among their fellow doctors. They are mostly detached from the patients as they "rotate" through different positions weekly or monthly, just keeping up with the algorithms, guidelines and protocols the hospital tells them to follow. They believe that most of their lifetime clinical work is done by the time they have graduated residency. Even though they would have gained little training or experience at that point (relative to the training and experience they ultimately need), they are often immediately set up as teachers and directors of this or that. They believe the patient to be the responsibility of

anyone else but them, unless they are "on duty" at that moment. They cannot rely on their own clinical experience because it is so often lacking due to their being distracted by research pursuits, publishing pursuits, lecturing pursuits, social pursuits, meetings, etc., and so they often rely on looking things up on the internet – sometimes having no more clinical knowledge than the patient – and certainly having little insight into human nature and how it might contribute to the traditional doctor-patient relationship and contribute to the healing process.

8. Medical doctors of today are rarely dedicated to the extent that they let aspects of their personal life suffer to support their job as a physician or surgeon, especially if they are hospital-employed. There are now laws and regulations in place that pretend to protect the health and safety of medical doctors in training so that they do not have to work too hard or for too long so that they can spend more time reading and studying at the expense of learning advanced skills of patient care and surgical technique, and at the expense of patient continuity of care and quality of care. It has all gone soft and weak of mind and body. It results in diminished competency of medical doctors and lower quality of care for patients.

9. Medical doctors of today have abrogated their leadership roles in their communities and in society and so society is in decay. They willingly or unwillingly comply with reporting private information about their patients to governmental agencies and willingly or unwillingly comply with spending much of their time doing data entry into electronic databases which serve to benefit a myriad of third party entities (but not necessarily the patient) – this behavior may have sinister consequences in the future.

10. Many medical doctors of today do not understand that the practice of medicine and surgery is an art that requires a mature and wise understanding of human nature superimposed on the application of scientific knowledge and technology – and would prefer to argue against that concept. There is this misguided concept of "evidence-based-medicine" which seeks to subvert and conceal wisdom and clinical experience in exchange for an academic-imposed process whereby flawed and biased publications are cited as "evidence" for how to diagnose and treat a patient. This ignores the fact that such publications have strict inclusion and exclusion criteria that render it impossible to expand the application of the data to all patients or to any individual patient. This ignores the fact that what is good for 63% of patients in one study may not be good for any given patient in the real world. This ignores the fact that these studies are broadly interpreted in an all-or-none approach as if the practice of medicine can be reduced to a recipe. This ignores the fact that the studies that are chosen for publication are sometimes chosen through a biased process based on personal opinions and the desire to manipulate and control information. This ignores the fact that creative statisticians can manipulate data, under most circumstances, to let it say whatever they want it to, albeit within some limits. The prevailing belief, like a religion now, is that if the government or the insurance company or the academic hospital can just form the right committee which can formulate the right algorithm for diagnosis and treatment, then this can be applied to any patient at any time and the health care system of the country will be perfect. This prevailing belief (given the infancy of current medical knowledge) is foolish.

Chapter Twenty Two:

The Ghost of American Health Care Future

1. If we continue on the current path which is transforming the American health care system, in the future, medical doctors will be governmental employees, drafted into service and placed geographically depending on the needs or desires of the government. There will be no medical schools, but there will be governmental training camps for the government medical algorithm-enforcers (this is what medical doctors, and all other "health care providers," will be called in the future).

2. Medical doctors of the future will be responsible for implementing the government's health care plan on the population. The government's health care plan will be coordinated with, and subsidiary to, a globalist agenda and a globalist governing body.

3. Surgeons of the future will be robots or else surgery may not be available for most people. However, there will be a carve-out for military personnel to get such treatment, and an additional carve out for upper echelon government officials to get the best treatment.

4. Ordinary citizens will get their health care by logging on to a governmental website. If their taxes are up to date, and there are no outstanding criminal or civil legal issues, then they will be allowed to proceed to the diagnostic module. They will enter

their list of symptoms. The governmental diagnostic algorithm will assign them a diagnosis, or they may be permitted to just "identify" with a diagnosis, and then a medication will be decided. The medication will be dispatched via drone from a government pharmacy. The drone will drop off the medication at the patient's location.

5. There will be no costs to any patient for any medical services, it will all be covered by taxes.

6. There will be no malpractice lawsuits or claims allowed because citizens will never be permitted to sue or make claim against the government even if there are terrible errors. However, if any patient pursues health care outside of the governmental system, then that will be considered criminal activity for both the patient and the unauthorized health care practitioner – this will warrant jail time and financial consequences for both.

7. Hospitals will still exist but will be governmental facilities. If the care that is needed goes beyond simple measures such as utilization of available medications or utilization of available robotic surgical technology, then the patient will be left to die, or survive on his own, due to the potential costs. However, the government will reserve the right to engage in euthanasia.

8. Once a health care provider has been chosen and trained by the government, he cannot choose another profession unless given special permission by the government through a complicated, lengthy and difficult process. If any health care provider does not perform according to governmental standards or comply with direct orders, it will be considered criminal

activity, especially after reprimands and retraining efforts, then incarceration will be the consequences.

9. There will be a secret squadron of medical doctors and medical researchers, for the purpose of providing state of the art medical care for the upper echelons of governmental personnel, for the purpose of developing biotechnological warfare and defense against biotechnological warfare and for the purpose of serving the government in any other way that the government dictates.

10. Social engineering will take place on such a scale that it will pervade every aspect of every community. Every citizen will have every aspect of their existence continuously recorded in multimedia by the government, including every keystroke they enter on any device. No citizen will be allowed to have a name, only a government-assigned number. There will be no traditional families allowed. The government will decide who can procreate with whom and at what time. The biological parents will have no control over, or involvement with, their offspring. The government will engage in genetic engineering as it so desires. The government will decide the racial ratio of the country, and likely decide to blend the races so there will be no clear racial distinction. The government will decide the number of same-gender-attraction individuals allowable, and may assign anyone into a same-gender relationship, even against their will, if it so desires. Alternatively, the government may decide to exterminate all individuals discovered with same-gender attraction, if it so desires. The government will decide the balance of gender, and may decide to medically change anyone's gender at any time, even against their will, if it so desires. The government will decide when and if to abort a pregnancy. Drinking water will have a contraceptive that requires an antidote

that only the government will have, and having a private water well will be unlawful. There will be no laws against rape of any kind; the word "rape" will be deleted from the English language. The government will control the upbringing and education of all infants and children. The government will decide the occupation of each individual, in collusion with corporate giants. Private enterprise will be allowable but only by collusion with government. Business and personal income will be heavily taxed, and there will be absolute limits on wealth. There will be no private land or private property ownership; all land or space will be rented from the government.

Chapter Twenty Three:

The Ghost of American Health Care Possible Future

1. If we allow clinical allopathic medical doctors to govern the path of health care, allow a more natural evolution, take the lawyers, politicians, academics, insurance companies, corporate giants, lobbyists and the like out of the process, we will wind up with a system which will be far more successful and satisfying for medical doctors and patients – and much less costly. These future medical doctors will dedicate many years of their early lives serving as apprentices to more experienced and competent clinical medical doctor mentors. These mentors will take care of patients both in the community setting and in the hospital setting – but they will be independent of hospital and academic control. The hospitals will be like athletic arenas; the arena owners don't get involved with managing the sports teams, and so the hospital owners won't get involved with telling the doctors how to practice medicine or perform surgery or keep their medical records. Most medical doctors will wisely avoid being involved in research and academia until they have had at least two decades of real-world hands-on experience taking care of patients – most will avoid it forever. During their training and subsequent practice, medical doctors will know how to protect themselves from risk of harm, at the same time still serving to take care of patients in dangerous circumstances. All for the sake of becoming experts in the practice of clinical medicine or surgery in the service of their patients.

2. Upon completion of medical school and subsequent clinical apprenticeships, medical doctors of this future will be indisputable experts dedicated to the clinical practice of medicine and surgery in the pursuit of excellence. The concepts of academic, hospital-based "internship" and "residency" and "fellowship" training programs will no longer exist. Medical doctors in training will learn how to become clinicians by working as apprentices with clinical medical doctor mentors rather than by wasting valuable time and resources in academia and research. Hence, the training process timeline, in most cases, will be substantially reduced, and will result in a substantially higher percentage of competent medical doctors practicing clinical medicine and surgery. Additionally, as they mature throughout their careers, medical doctors will be able to expand or transition their expertise without being limited by fellowship and board requirements, especially as needed in underserved communities. They will be fluid in their skills and services. For example, a neurologist can become a pediatrician, a gynecologist can become a psychiatrist, pursuant to their evolving talents and the evolving needs of any community.

Clinical medical doctors will constitute a substantial proportion of the teaching positions at medical schools, and they will be paid by the medical schools for their teaching. Ph.D.s will still play an integral part of the initial basic sciences education and training of medical students, and will still dominate in laboratory medical research, but they will gain additional dominance over clinical medical research. We will create the concept of a clinical Ph.D. expressly for the purpose of clinical medical research projects and clinical trials. Rather than wasting the valuable and rare M.D. slots on researchers, we will draw from the vast overpopulation of Ph.D.s to take the place of the misguided "M.D.-Ph.D." concept. This will enable so much more research without drawing from the severely underpopulated pool of M.D.s which are desperately needed to provide clinical care. The time line of medical school will be shortened from four years down to three continuous years.

There will be no more board certification entities and hence no maintenance of certification programs, but there will be robust continuing medical education programs mostly run by clinical medical doctor mentors teamed with clinical Ph.D. researchers.

3. The physicians and surgeons of this future will be so dedicated and so busy taking care of people because they will be protected from needlessly burdensome legislative issues, legal issues, regulatory issues, academic issues, research issues, insurance issues or any issues outside of improving their excellence in the practice of the art of medicine and surgery – because the health care system (on local, state and federal levels) will be run by clinical medical doctors and not by lawyers, politicians, academics, researchers, insurance companies, corporate giants, lobbyists and the like. Research will be funded primarily by private companies in collaboration with academia so that funding will not be subject to the fluctuations caused by taxpayers and politicians.

4. The physicians and surgeons of this future will be appropriately respected and appreciated for their indispensable contribution to society, and, more than money, these medical doctors will value their role in society and receive their greatest satisfaction from helping others.

5. The physicians and surgeons of this future will wisely understand the balance of financial compensation: they will charge a fair price commensurate with their needs and abilities, and commensurate with what the market will bear. This future medical doctor will balance his practice with a cross section of patients in such a way that he will remain financially solvent. No governmental agency, legislative regulation or insurance company policy will dictate what the doctor can or cannot charge or collect. Medical doctors will take business courses in medical school and will be trained, by their mentors, regarding how to run a successful business.

The medical doctors themselves will decide if they want to participate in electronic health records or use paper charts or some other system or some combination – there will be no standard controlled by government. The medical doctors themselves will decide how to write their notes based on personal preferences combined with professional standards tailored to their practices and their patient populations – these will not be micromanaged by governmental bureaucratic regulations, hospital administrators, litigation expectations or insurance company policies.

Insurance companies will be involved with reimbursing the patient not the medical doctor. No medical doctor will deal directly with any insurance company (commercial or governmental) for payments, or be subjected to their health care dictates of any kind, due to the conflicts of interest and due to the financial inefficiencies. Health care Insurance companies will be allowed to provide payments and policies that cross state lines to foster free-market competition, to enable larger participation pools and hence to enable lower rates and improved services.

The Ghost of American Health Care Possible Future

With new legislation, insurance companies will no longer enjoy the apparent exemption from antitrust or anti-collusion regulations and so will no longer be able to collude in price-fixing schemes.

The better doctors (defined as being more clinically experienced and better able to achieve good outcomes for their patients) will be more sought out and hence more highly compensated.

Health care costs will be dramatically less than they are today, but medical doctors will have a higher quality of life and patients will be served faster and more successfully.

The governmental programs of Medicare and Medicaid will be recognized as having been unconstitutional. They will be one hundred percent converted to a defined contribution program rather than a defined benefit program. This defined contribution will be a sum of money paid by the government as an annual stipend to each American citizen. This stipend must be used to pay for a commercial health insurance policy. It will be mandatory to purchase health care insurance in order to receive the stipend. The stipend may be more or less than the cost of the annual policy, but it will be up to the individual to decide which policy to purchase (a more or less expensive one). Couples and family members can combine their stipends to purchase couple or family policies. This program will be funded by payroll taxes. However, the beneficiaries will be every United States citizen, instead of being limited by age or income level or disability. Converting these governmental programs in this way will help every person to become insured, but will block the current government micro-management of, and interference with, the doctor-patient relationship. Converting these governmental programs in this way will save the federal and state governments countless billions of dollars in their budgets annually. Converting these governmental programs in this way will extinguish the obsolete and unsustainable burden of employer-based health care. Converting these governmental programs in this way will eliminate fraud and abuse issues against government funds. Converting these governmental programs in this way will enable the government to increase the applicable payroll tax (employers will be happy to pay it because they will no longer be paying for employee health insurance and so will have a windfall surplus) at the same time the governmental payouts will decrease substantially and perhaps this mega surplus could be used to help convert the current Social Security pyramid scheme to a fully funded retirement account (and even enable residual beneficiary designation upon death) – hence additionally contributing to the health of the American society.

If there are concerns about high costs of insurance to the elderly or to the chronically ill, then the solutions will be in the free market combined with minimally invasive state regulations, not in the federal government. Furthermore, health insurance policies will not be limited to annual policies, and will be made multi-year term, or life-long, similar to life insurance policies.

Additionally, pre-tax programs such as health savings accounts [HSAs] or a flex spending accounts [FSAs] will be expanded, not diminished or deleted, and perpetually allowed annual roll-over – especially as a means for patients to pay for health care costs prior to being reimbursed by insurance. Furthermore, nursing home care will be more commonly covered under appropriate insurance policies rather than under Medicaid.

The Ghost of American Health Care Possible Future

6. At this future time it will be understood that medical doctors are only human and the art of the practice of medicine or surgery is not an exact science, and doctors are not infallible machines, and doctors do not cause illnesses or injuries, and doctors do not make the dysfunctional lifestyle decisions that often cause patients to become chronically ill, and doctors do not decide the genetic disposition of patients, and doctors do not control the patients' compliance with treatments, and doctors have no control over the limits of medical knowledge and technology. And so doctors will not be liable for the outcomes unless there is fraud or criminal activity perpetrated.

However, this future medical doctor will see the doctor-patient interaction as one that reveals problems that need to be solved as a team. The team will consist of the patient and the doctor with support from the patient's family and friends and additional support from the doctor's staff. The patient's problems will become the doctor's problems. The doctor-patient interaction will no longer be an occasion to merely preach advice, but will require the medical doctor to function on an as-yet-unseen level of influence whereby the patient will be successful in achieving dramatic lifestyle changes and in achieving timely compliance with the treatment plan – all leading to an optimal outcome for the patient. Clinical research will focus more on how the doctor can help the patient truly achieve an improved lifestyle. Another important area of future clinical research will focus on helping medical doctors maintain a healthy lifestyle themselves while they perform at a high level of dedication to their patients.

The patient won't need a health care team consisting of a team of doctors (each partially incompetent – requiring a bunch of them to coordinate their efforts together to achieve minimal competence), as is the current trend. Instead the patient will be on his own team and will take personal responsibility for his own problems and will have one abundantly competent doctor as his teammate personally and professional devoted to an optimal outcome.

If there is a poor outcome for a patient because his human medical doctor made a human error, then there will be a no-fault insurance program – managed and funded by this future American health care system (funds built up by recurring charges to all medical doctors, all hospitals, all pharmaceutical companies and all biomedical technology companies), overseen by a consortium of medical doctors and patient representatives and financial experts (no lawyers need to be involved) – to help urgently finance the ongoing care of this patient.

7. Medical doctors of this future will maintain an adversarial relationship with hospitals, medical centers and health care organizations – understanding that they are the ultimate advocates for what is best for the patient and for themselves, and understanding that the hospitals, medical centers and health care organizations focus is primarily on financial health over patient health. They will be independent practitioners or in private group practices, but almost never will they allow themselves to be employees of the hospital, medical center or health care organization due to the serious conflict of interest that will then be set up – although they will partner with hospitals as necessary to maintain continuity of care for their patients. Hospitals will abandon the archaic and unhealthy concept of "on-call" and will adopt a subcontractor shift program to ensure the health of the community's doctors as well as the health of the community's

patients. Every night, weekend and holiday in every hospital, there will be seasoned experienced medical doctors and surgeons onsite to serve patients, instead of just trainees available (with the seasoned doctors and surgeons, available by phone, sleeping at home after a long day of service) as it is currently configured. Hospitals will be owned and administered by medical doctors and surgeons who remain engaged in clinical practice. There will be no more regional mini monopolies of hospital conglomerates. With new legislation, medical doctors that are employees of hospitals, medical centers or large health care organizations will be entitled to unionize or otherwise engage in collective bargaining. Certificate of need regulations will be abolished as they promote monopolies and restrict competition, and so new innovative facilities will sprout up all over the place to improve choices and quality of medical care while reducing costs.

8. Medical doctors of this future will be dedicated to the extent that most aspects of their personal life will be configured such as to support their vocation – their calling – as a physician or surgeon. They will have the abilities and support in place to take on greater aspects of commitment to the successful outcomes for their patients. Medical doctors who are unwilling to do this will avoid or leave the practice of medicine and make way for those who are willing.

9. Medical doctors of this future will play stable leadership roles in their communities and their communities will wisely include medical doctors in improving and maintaining community health.

Allopathic medical doctors, privately practicing as clinical physicians and surgeons, will be recognized and valued as the national treasures that they are, and as such, will be protected and defended by society.

Clinical allopathic medical doctors will be in charge of all boards of public health and boards of medicine in each state and territory of the United States of America. All other health care providers or practitioners of every type imaginable will fall under their jurisdiction – no longer will there be parallel boards or separate governance constructs for each type of clinical practitioner or health care provider. True allopathic medical doctors will set the standards and thresholds for clinical care privileges and licensure regarding all participants in the clinical health care world.

10. Medical doctors of this future will understand that the practice of medicine and surgery is an art that requires a mature and wise understanding of human nature superimposed on the application of scientific knowledge and technology. The outcome will have just as much to do with the way the doctor interacts with the patient and the patient's family as it does with identifying the correct diagnosis or prescribing the correct medication or performing the appropriate surgical procedure. It will be understood that the human body has the inherent ability to heal itself, and the doctor is there to facilitate that natural healing process.

Chapter Twenty Four:

Summary Suggestions for the American Health Care System

1. In this book I have tried to present an insider's perspective of the current state of the American health care system in the year 2016. Yes, my perspective is biased based on the point of view of an allopathic medical doctor; however, without allopathic medical doctor physicians and surgeons, there would be no health care system. It seems that the voices of allopathic medical doctors have been relegated to last place in recent years, most likely due to their own lack of effective participation in regulatory processes, and due to the aggressiveness of all the other voices trying to take control. But there is a direct correlation between ignoring the allopathic medical doctors and the destruction of the American health care system. I am not advocating to ignore the voices of all the other participants in the health care system, but those other voices must be tertiary to the voices of the allopathic medical doctors and their patients. Below I summarize the most significant suggestions presented in this book.

2. To my fellow medical doctors: Focus on the practice of clinical medicine. Minimize your academic, research and publishing pursuits (at least until later in your careers when you will make more meaningful contributions). Focus on your patients. Understand that you do not work for your hospital, your medical school, your academic department or the government. You work for your patients. When you pursue CME courses each year,

expand the spectrum of your study to include topics outside your area of specialty. If feasible, expand the services you provide in your practice to better serve the needs of your community rather than restrict your services out of personal interest or convenience. Take a leadership role in your community and be active in your state medical societies and professional associations. Contribute generously to lobbying efforts that benefit the medical profession. Become politically involved on local, state and federal levels.

Join with your fellow medical doctors to take back stewardship of the American health care system before it deteriorates any further. Abandon hospital employment positions, abandon academic positions and get back to private practice. Stop quarreling amongst yourselves over trivial ego-driven issues. Consider the broader societal consequences. Understand that as you fight your mole-hill battles, a multitude of outside forces are gaining inappropriate but absolute control over the medical profession. United we thrive and save the American health care system. Divided we suffer and American patients suffer.

Consider dis-enrolling from the Medicare program, or at least stop enabling it and stop cooperating with it. It is a system that abuses medical doctors year after year, with the abuse getting worse each year. Most medical doctors continue to take the abuse year after year like prostitutes for their payments. It is only when all medical doctors abandon the Medicare program that Medicare will begin to do the right thing for medical doctors and patients. However, medical doctors must never abandon their patients. Continue to pursue excellence in service to your patients; keep this as your focus.

Summary Suggestions for the American Health Care System

Do NOT allow Medicare, commercial health insurers, lawyers, hospital administrators or any third party dictate how you practice medicine or perform surgery. Do NOT allow Medicare, commercial health insurers, lawyers, hospital administrators or any third party dictate how you write or store your patient records – do it in a way that enables you to practice efficiently and effectively without incurring undue time consumption or financial burden.

Consider discontinuing participation the board certification process, at least until board monopolies are busted up, until certification processes are more practical, until certification is made life long, and until the ability to add additional certifications is reasonably achievable in a short period of time. Discontinue participation in any maintenance of certification process.

Take the oath presented in Chapter Two of this book.

3. To medical students, interns and residents: Dismiss the myth that you need to focus on research in order to be a successful medical doctor. The opposite is true. Spend less time with exam preparation and more time with hands on clinical patient care involvement. Don't waste your training years reading so much; focus on doing! Seek out mentors and apprenticeship type relationships with experienced clinical physicians and surgeons; these more experienced doctors will be very receptive to having you around. When you finish your training, get out of the hospitals and academic institutes, go into the private practice setting. It is in the private practice setting where the real learning will take place (although, understandably, some types of surgeons and emergency room doctors will need to work in hospitals exclusively). If you stay at the academic hospitals after your

training, your growth and experience will be severely retarded, and you will never reach your full potential. I encourage you to practice in rural and underserved areas. This is where you are needed most and where you will grow best.

4. To medical schools: Find ways to make medical education more efficient, of shorter duration, of lower cost, more focused on the clinical practice of medicine and surgery and abandon any focus on research for the medical students. Include education and training in business, practice management, marketing as well as legal and legislative matters. Abandon the "M.D.-Ph.D." concept, and save the M.D. degree slots only for those who want to be directly involved with patient care. Initiate a clinical-Ph.D. pathway for focus on biomedical clinical research and clinical trials. Consider becoming independent from any university system: stand-alone private medical school education has the best potential to be more innovative, adaptive and free from conflicts of interest.

5. To hospitals, medical centers, major health care organizations and academic facilities: Abandon the obsession of employing physicians and surgeons, keep it to a minimum. Allow private practices to contract as individuals or groups to cover inpatient services. Move toward shift work with seasoned experienced medical doctors and surgeons onsite at all times for inpatient issues, discontinue the "on-call" concept, and get out of the outpatient business. Abandon academic constructs in medical and surgical practices. The constructs of instructors, assistant professors, associate professors, full professors, division chiefs, department chairs, etc., are all failed artificial constructs in the context of the clinical practice of medicine and surgery. Take leadership roles to redefine the practice of medicine and surgery

in the hospital setting. Discard the inhibiting militant hierarchical constructs and focus on serving patients and supporting doctors. As one example, try an annually (or every three years) rotating physician leadership program, or something to that effect, to achieve organization. Do not collude with insurance companies and governmental bodies against the doctors and patients, instead support the doctors and patients against intrusions by the insurance companies and governmental bodies. Abandon EHRs that are not focused on improving the doctor-patient interaction, and don't make a specific brand of EHR use mandatory on all affiliated doctors, unless exclusively for inpatient care.

6. To any and all organizations, institutions, governmental agencies and regulatory bodies that are involved in medical and surgical internships, residencies, fellowship and board certification programs: Take leadership roles and expand these programs beyond the limitations of hospitals and academic medical centers, and do away with the concept of board certification. Partnerships with private practice mentors for apprenticeship positions may be more efficient, effective, take less time and provide alternative means of financing such training to spare the taxpayers. The concept of the federal government paying for training programs can be eliminated entirely. Furthermore, as medical doctors mature throughout their careers, they must be allowed to expand or transition their expertise without being limited by residency, fellowship and board certification constraints, especially as needed in underserved communities. They must be allowed to be fluid in their skills and services, through the proposed establishment of mentoring and apprenticeship models. For example, a neurologist must be allowed to expand to also practice pediatrics,

a gynecologist must be allowed to expand to also practice psychiatry, etc., pursuant to their evolving talents and the evolving needs of any community.

7. To professional medical associations: Abandon the undue burden of board certification, at least until board monopolies are busted up, until certification processes are more practical, until certification is made life long, and until the ability to add additional certifications is reasonably achievable in a short period of time. Abandon all maintenance of certification [MOC] programs. To health care insurers and hospital credentialing organizations: Discontinue the requirements of board certification and MOC – accept residency graduation and medical licensing as more than sufficient. To professional medical associations: Discontinue accepting the annual Medicare manipulations. Stop teaching your members how to jump through the new Medicare hoops each year. Instead, tell your members to ignore all Medicare mandates, tell them to suffer the financial penalties. After a few years, Medicare payments will be so low, due to the accumulated penalties, then all medical doctors will have no problem abandoning the Medicare program. Medicare must not be allowed the authority to tell medical doctors how to practice medicine. It was intended to be an insurance policy program. It is only when all medical doctors abandon the Medicare program that Medicare will begin to do the right thing for medical doctors and patients.

8. To health care insurance companies: Discontinue the practice of medicine. Discontinue telling medical doctors and surgeons what they can and cannot do. If you can't afford to do what the doctors want and what the patients need, then get out of the business. If applicable, discontinue collusion with each other and

Summary Suggestions for the American Health Care System

with CMS in price-fixing schemes. Be more efficient. Focus more on serving the patients and the doctors. Discontinue payments for anything other than allopathic health care under the direction of allopathic medical doctors. Abandon the artificial construct of having doctors "in network." Reconfigure your payment plans to pay for any allopathic medical doctor's service, even across state lines, if the doctor is willing to see your covered patients for your rates. Do not restrict your patients against seeing the allopathic medical doctor of their choice. Also, standardize and publish your rates, do not have multiple secretive rates that discriminate against some doctors over others.

Commercial health care insurance companies must deal directly with the patients and not at all with the medical doctors or hospitals. The concept of using pre-tax health savings accounts [HSAs] or flex spending accounts [FSAs] must be expanded for the benefit of patients to be able to cover medical doctor and hospital costs prior to receiving reimbursements from insurance. Individual health insurance policies must not be limited to annual policies, and could be made multi-year term, or life-long, similar to life insurance policies. Coverage of nursing home costs must be incorporated into insurance policy options.

9. To pharmaceutical companies and biomedical technology companies: Keep up the good work you do coming up with cures, treatments and devices that help us diagnose and treat our patients, thank you. Be more efficient. Lobby for a substitute to the patent system. Seek a new category of some hybrid between trademark and trade secret for your products so that the protection is indefinite. Seek modification of the FDA's methods and regulations so that you can get products to market faster, at less cost and so the FDA will share or assume product liability.

10.   To lawyers and legislators: Discontinue the current constructs of medical malpractice lawsuits and pharmaceutical and biomedical technology product liability lawsuits.   Convert these to no-fault insurance claims situations whereby the harmed patients will quickly receive more money and timely care. At the same time, this new system will substantially reduce costs to the health care system.   It will put health care trial lawyers out of business.   Their litigating activity, arguably, has not improved health care, but has driven up costs and wasted valuable time; it's time to stop it. This program can be funded either by a payroll tax or by annually recurring prorated charges to all medical doctors, hospitals, pharmaceutical companies and biomedical technology companies. Additionally, Individuals must be enabled to privately purchase such insurance coverage.

11.   To governmental agencies and elected representatives: Eliminate the Medicaid system and change the current Medicare system from one of defined benefits for the elderly to one of defined contribution to each citizen.   Converting these governmental programs in this way will help every person to become insured, but will block the current government micro-management of, and interference with, the doctor-patient relationship.   Converting these governmental programs in this way will save the federal and state governments countless billions of dollars in their budgets annually, will extinguish the obsolete and unsustainable burden of employer-based health care, and will eliminate fraud and abuse issues against governmental funds. Converting these governmental programs in this way will enable the government to increase the applicable payroll tax as employers will be happy to pay more because they will no longer be paying for employee health insurance and so will have a

windfall surplus and at the same time the governmental payouts will decrease substantially. If there are concerns about high costs of insurance to the elderly or to the chronically ill, then the solutions will be in the free market combined with minimally invasive state regulations, not in the federal government.

Expand health savings accounts [HSAs] and flex spending account [FSAs] for the benefit of patients to be able to cover medical costs directly payable to medical doctors and hospitals. The ability to fund such accounts must be more liberal, the ability to invest the deposits must be allowed (with no tax consequences) and annual roll-over of funds must be perpetual. Insurance reimbursements to the patients can then go back into these accounts, with no tax consequences, once received.

Large conglomerate hospital mini monopolies need to be busted up, and certificate of need regulations must be abolished in states that still have such regulations. New entities must have no barriers to compete with the well-established facilities: this will accelerate innovation, increase choices and drive prices down

Legislate that the federal government can no longer provide spousal benefits of any kind or define marriage. Spousal benefits must be converted to couple benefits. Every single adult citizen must be entitled to designate one other adult as their coupled beneficiary. Government must get out of the marriage business, and all people must be treated equally, including single people who are still being treated unequally under the law in violation of their Constitutional rights.

12. To the states' boards of medicine: Take a greater leadership role, working closely with clinical allopathic medical doctors, to be better stewards and guardians of the American health care

system. Do not allow alternative practitioners to usurp leadership of the health care system or to create parallel regulatory systems. Take over as masters of credentialing so that medical doctors will come to you as the only centralized repository of all their credentialing information, to be updated by them only as needed, and to be distributed to all others (hospitals, insurance companies, etc.) as needed and as authorized. Establish simple and rapid licensing reciprocity for all other states' medical licensees; this will expedite your ability to recruit to underserved areas.

13. To any and all who will listen and understand: It is time to restore free-market forces back into the American health care system. It is time for medical doctors and patients to deal directly with one another with no third party in between to control health care decisions or health care pricing.

14. To any and all who will listen and understand: It is time to increase society's mental health resources. It is time for a one hundred fold increase in mental health clinicians and services, and a one hundred fold increase in mental health facility capacity.

15. To politicians: Serve the people of your districts and states, minimize lobbyists' influence over you if it is not in the absolute best interest of your constituents. Remember the idealistic reasons you went into "public service" in the first place before you were intoxicated by money and seduced by the illusion of power. Understand that power is best measured by the control you have over yourself not by the control you have over other people. Begin the process of enacting the 28th Amendment of the United States Constitution, regarding the Right to Freedom of Health Care, as proposed in Chapter Seven of this book.

Summary Suggestions for the American Health Care System

16. To patients: Reach out to your state and federal representatives and demand a better health care system. Demand one that is focused on supporting medical doctors and patients. Demand that health care decisions be reserved exclusively for the allopathic medical doctors and their patients, and not in the hands of the federal government or commercial insurance companies.

If you enjoy alternative practitioners who limit themselves to their trades, then be supportive of them to the extent that they are truly supportive of your care, but be cautious of being used primarily for their monetary gain. Avoid alternative practitioners such as naturopaths, homeopaths, herbalists, acupuncturists, chiropractors, massage therapists and faith healers who try to practice allopathic medicine or try to order or perform allopathic medical tests or procedures – none of them have the appropriate knowledge, experience or appropriate skill to do so. You might be harmed and a substantial amount of money might be needlessly drained from the health care system (or from you).

Avoid hospital-employed or academic medical doctors and surgeons. Instead seek out private practice medical doctors and surgeons – don't be afraid to ask. Supporting private practice clinical allopathic medical doctors and surgeons is one of the best ways to thwart the destructive forces ruining our health care system today. Avoid academic or so called teaching hospitals wherever possible, better to utilize community or non-teaching hospitals for higher quality and more personalized care.

Instruct all of your doctors to keep your personal medical records in a system that is not online or at least that is not a "shared" electronic system – to keep it private between you and your doctor and restrict access to any third party unless by your authority in writing. Provide these instructions to your doctor in writing and hold him accountable if he fails to do so.

Seek out allopathic medical doctors that focus on clinical medicine and surgery (as opposed to those involved with academia, teaching and research). Seek out those who are experienced, who are wise, who are attentive, who spend sufficient time with you, who educate you and who effectively communicate with you. I suggest you print out Chapter Two of this book and ask your doctor to take that oath. Those who do, if they are sincere, are likely to be the most helpful to you.

Warning: There is a significant and growing shortage of clinical allopathic medical doctors in America today. Most medical doctors no longer accept Medicaid-type insurance (even though enrollment in Medicaid-type insurance is skyrocketing). In a few years it is likely that most doctors will no longer accept Medicare insurance. Medical doctors are being subjected to ever increasing unreasonable demands and regulations which contribute to burnout, early retirement, quitting and even suicide. New governmental laws and regulations regarding health care have made things much worse for doctors and patients – the full effect of these laws and regulations will be unfolding more profoundly in the coming years. If nothing is done to stop this, then the remaining functional aspects of the American health care system will be destroyed, and the doctor shortage will become an extreme acute crisis. Medical doctors are under attack from every angle imaginable and they just cannot take it anymore.

Do your part, play an active role to the best of your ability – be an advocate for yourself and for your medical doctor. Help make the American health care system great again.

About the Author:

Dr. Warinner received his Bachelor of Science degree in pre-medical studies from the University of Notre Dame in Indiana. He studied biomedical engineering at the Cooper Union Engineering School in Manhattan, New York. He received his M.D. degree at New York Medical College in Valhalla, New York. He did general surgery internship and neurosurgery residency training at New York University Medical Center and Bellevue Hospital in Manhattan. He spent a semester training at the Centre Hospitalier Sainte-Anne in Paris, France. He completed his Neurology residency training at the Harvard Medical School combined Massachusetts General Hospital and Brigham and Women's Hospital program. He spent time training at The Neurological Institute of Mental Health and Neurological Surgery [NIMHANS] in Bangalore, India, and surrounding facilities. During both residencies he served at three different VA medical centers. He did an additional internship in internal medicine at Sound Shore Medical Center in New Rochelle, New York. He did fellowship training in clinical neurophysiology at Harvard Brigham and Women's Hospital. It is through the neuromuscular division and the electrodiagnostic laboratory at Brigham and Women's Hospital that he maintained an academic affiliation and part-time teaching position for more than a decade. It was there that he was made the inaugural Director of Sports Neurology and established their Sports Concussion Clinic. He currently maintains multiple hospital affiliations in the Boston area. He also maintains an adjunct teaching position at New York Medical College. He achieved board certification by the American Board of Psychiatry and Neurology and achieved subspecialty board certification in the areas of Electrodiagnostic Medicine and Neuromuscular

Medicine. He has since achieved subsequent maintenance of certification requirements.

Dr. Warinner has spent time at the National Institutes of Health assisting in neuroscience research and he has been involved in clinical research serving as a principal investigator. For decades, he has been involved in private charitable fundraising for neuroscience research. He regularly provides medical educational presentations and webinars for medical schools, hospitals, professional medical organizations and pharmaceutical companies. He has had numerous appearances on television and radio regarding medical commentary. He has been involved in leadership positions and has provided educational presentations at the American Academy of Neurology and at the American Association of Neuromuscular and Electrodiagnostic Medicine. He serves as Chair of the Electrodiagnostic Laboratory Accreditation program. He serves as the Massachusetts State Liaison on a committee which periodically meets with U.S. senatorial and congressional offices to educate political leaders about quality of medical care and about fighting against health care fraud. He has served as expert medical witness on numerous civil and criminal cases. He has been involved with helping the FBI root out and prosecute health care fraud and he has worked with commercial health insurance companies in health care fraud investigations. He has been involved in the creation of medically-related state legislation.

Dr. Warinner is licensed as a medical doctor and has practiced medicine in three states. He is a licensed ringside physician and current Chair of the Medical Advisory Board for the Massachusetts State Athletic Commission. He serves as a part-time prison neurologist. He is medical director of a private multispecialty group practice serving the suburban community west of Boston. This facility is considered one of the most comprehensive clinical neurophysiology laboratories in the country, with particular expertise in sports neurology. Although he works with professional athletes, Olympic athletes, collegiate athletes, television and radio personalities, writers, artists and the like, he mostly serves ordinary adults and children from the community. He focuses his practice on medical and surgical issues of a neurological nature. These neurological problems include head trauma, concussions, Parkinson's disease, Alzheimer's disease, dementia, multiple sclerosis, brain tumors, stroke, cerebral aneurysms, neurological infections, muscular dystrophy, peripheral neuropathy, peripheral nerve injury in sports, myasthenia gravis, myopathy, mitochondrial disorders, spinal cord and nerve root problems, Lyme disease, sleep disorders, headaches, seizures, epilepsy, psychological or psychiatric conditions and more.

Dr. Warinner plans to continue serving patients in the community, mentoring fellow medical doctors, volunteering to fight medical fraud, advocating for the preservation of private practice, advising state and federal governmental bodies on improving quality of patient care and working overall to shape a better future for the American health care system. Join his effort to make the American health care system great again.

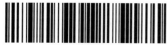

Made in the USA
Middletown, DE
24 March 2017